Better Health: Happier Living

53 Ways to Dramatically Improve Your Health and Well-Being

David Klein

Better Health: Happier Living. 53 Ways to Dramatically Improve Your Health and Well-Being. Copyright © David Klein, 2019. All rights reserved. Printed in the United States of America. No part of this book may be copied or reproduced in any manner whatsoever without written permission, except in the case of brief quotations embodied in critical articles and reviews. Please use the contact information below.

ISBN: 9781095399712
Edited by David Klein
Cover Design by PixelStudios
Mediterranean Pyramid Image: Oldways, www.oldwayspt.org

v 1.13

DISCLAIMER: This book is intended as an educational tool only and is not intended to provide personal medical advice. Rather, it's a book that teaches the principles of sound nutrition and lifestyle enhancements. If you have a medical issue or are looking for medical advice, or if you believe that you need to make dietary changes to improve your health, it is recommended that you consult with a qualified physician.

david@davidkleinwriting.com
www.davidkleinwriting.com

Acknowledgements

This book has been written for all those who want to enjoy good health, but who have been plied with so much misinformation that they don't really know what to do. Some of that misinformation was likely health-damaging, and it may have been very costly. May you find the pathway to better health through the simple, logical, and tried-and-true health methods discussed in this book.

A special thanks to Vani Hari, otherwise known as the Food Babe. Vani has a passion for good, clean, natural food, and she's made a career of helping to expose the many chemical and otherwise harmful ingredients that are routinely added to our foods. She has blazed a trail right to the headquarters of companies that are among the biggest offenders, and she's persuaded many to remove hazardous ingredients from their offerings. We all owe Vani a big thank you for that. So here's my thank you: Vani, thank you for having the intelligence, the wisdom, the courage, the class, the love, and the energy to make a change. I love reading your books and watching your videos. You are excellent at what you do. And your work has clearly paid you with personal rewards. Your appearance and your personality wonderfully radiate with a healthy glow . . . you truly walk the walk.

And a special thanks to Dr. Alan Christianson, affectionately known as "Dr. C." by many. Dr. C. is my favorite health and nutrition writer ever. He is brilliant, he totally "gets it," and he lovingly and enthusiastically shares his treasure of knowledge with others.

Dr. C. has a wonderful gift of possessing a huge wealth of knowledge and understanding of all matters health and nutrition. And he possesses a wonderful gift of taking all that information and explaining it in the most delightful, easy-to-understand, and easy-to-apply manner.

One more thing about getting to know Dr. C.s work . . . it may cost you some money. But this is money you'll delight in spending. So many who apply what Dr. C. teaches not only dramatically improve their health but also lose unwanted pounds in the process. That means, of course, some newer, smaller-sized clothing for the new-and-improved slimmer and more dapper you. Not a bad deal at all!

And thanks to others who work in the field of health and nutrition who also "get it," meaning that they have learned to think outside the box and see health and nutrition for what it really is, and then have courageously used that knowledge to blaze a path to better health for so many. Included in this special group are Diana Schwarzbein, T. Colin Campbell, Caldwell B. Esselstyn, Linda Khoshaba, Izabella Wentz, and so many others.

And finally, to my wife Rae. She's my favorite person in the world, and her outstanding qualities shine. I appreciate her more every year.

Practical wisdom is one of Rae's outstanding qualities. As an example, I'm a professional writer and she's a professional editor. She edited the first book I wrote, and she's smart enough to skillfully avoid another team effort. (Husbands and wives, if you want a hilarious adventure, try having one write a book and the other edit that book. Decision making time is a real hoot!)

And as I write in every book I've ever written, Rae Rae's the funniest person I've ever met. She finds and adds joy and humor to so many situations, and I'm deeply grateful for it.

Table of Contents

Introduction ix
How to Use this Book xi
Dietary Enhancements 1
   What to Eat 3
      1. "Eat the Rainbow" 3
      2. Eat Natural Foods 6
      3. Eat a Balance of Proteins, Fats, and Carbohydrates (The Three Macronutrients) 8
      4. Eat Living Foods 9
      5. Drink Plenty of Water 10
      6. Consider Eating Probiotics 11
      7. Consider Some Organic Foods 13
   What Not To Eat 15
      8. Don't Eat Refined Carbohydrates 15
      9. Don't Eat Bad Fats 17
      10. Don't Eat Chemicals 19
      11. Don't Eat Junk Food 21
      12. If You Have Food Allergies or Sensitivities, Avoid Those Foods 23
   When to Eat 27
      13. Don't Skip Breakfast, and Make it a High-Protein Meal ... 27
      14. Don't Eat More Than a Snack Late in the Evening 29
      15. Cycle Your Carbohydrates 30
   How to Eat 31
      16. Chew Your Food Thoroughly 31

17. Don't Overeat 33

18. How Much Should You Eat? 35

19. Keep Plenty of Healthful Foods on Hand; Keep Junk Foods out of the Home if Possible 37

20. If You Fall Off the Dietary Bandwagon, Get Right Back On 38

21. Is Fasting Really Healthy? An Alternative. 39

22. Avoid Fad Diets 42

23. Consider a High-Speed Blender 44

The Best Way to Eat, Recap 46

The World's Healthiest Diet 47

24. The Mediterranean Diet 47

25. Guidelines to Enhance the Mediterranean Diet 49

Additional Paths to Better Health 57

26. Exercise Your Body 59

27. Exercise Your Brain (Stay Mentally Sharp) 67

28. Maintain Your Proper Body Weight (And Shape) 73

29. Don't Lose Weight to Get Healthy; Get Healthy to Lose Weight 77

30. Get Adequate Sunlight 78

31. Enjoy Restful Sleep 81

32. Keep a Regular Routine if Possible 87

33. Accept Reality: And Deal With it Wisely 91

34. Be Your Own Person: Think for Yourself 92

35. Maintain Sound Oral Health 95

36. Have Fun: Immerse Yourself in a Hobby or Something Else You Love 97

37. Laugh Every Day—Maintain a Sense of Humor 100

38. Avoid Negative Thinking; Think Positive Thoughts 105
39. Build and Maintain a Large Circle of Friends 107
40. Don't Be a Perfectionist, Be Reasonable 109
41. Be Alert to Whatever May Drain Your Energy and Well-Being 111
42. Don't Be a Health Food Store Junk Food Junkie 113
43. Be Peaceful 115
44. Don't Blow Your Lid 116
45. Be Forgiving 118
46. Be Thankful 118
47. Be Generous 120
48. Be Loving 122
49. Don't Ignore the Whispers (Listen to Your Body) 123
50. Take Time For Yourself Every Day 124
51. Stay Educated About Health and Nutrition 126
52. View Your Health Like a Bank Account 127
53. Smile and Maintain a Happy Disposition 128

Index 131
Final Thoughts 149

Introduction

Are you satisfied with your health? Most people shouldn't be, because the health of the average person in the United States and around the world is abysmal. We are overweight, out of shape, overmedicated, hyper-tense, bloated, crammed with toxic chemicals, out of touch with the rhythms of natural living, and out of touch with ourselves.

Whose fault is it? There's lots of blame to go around. It starts, perhaps, with the huge amounts of misinformation that we've been taught, as well as with the huge amounts of good information that we have not been taught. Commercial advertisers have not helped, persuasively pushing "foods" whose sole health benefits are to the bank accounts of those who sell them. Many of us are confused and frustrated, and for good reason.

This book, *Better Health: Happier Living*, will correct this problem. I'll teach you what to eat, when to eat, how to eat, how to live in harmony with the rhythms of nature, how to live at peace with yourself and with others, and how to enjoy a more productive and fulfilling life.

There is nothing fanatical or "way out there" in this book. All of the methods of healthful living are time-proven and accepted by the vast majority of experts.

I never expected to write the following statement in a health book, but I feel a need to do so, as it's central to the theme of this book. That statement: I don't believe in evolution or that life came about by spontaneous accidents. Why is that central to the theme of this book?

Because it's clear to me that the human body and Earth were created as a beautiful match. Time and time again, it's been proven that the further we stray from nature, the more we get into trouble. For instance: Baby formula versus mother's milk? *It's not even close.*

Day shift work versus graveyard shift or swing shift? *Your body and mind know the answer. So does your social life.* Natural foods versus chemical substances with names like "butylated hydroxytoluene"? *If you can't spell it, don't eat it. It will likely make you sick.* Spring water versus aerated sugar/chemical water, otherwise known as soda? *Whoa.* Tobacco smoke inhaled in the lungs versus clean, oxygen-rich air. *Double whoa.* A balanced exercise program versus couch potato living? *Strength, stamina, flexibility, confidence, and stability versus being weak, overweight, oxygen-starved, and out-of-breath.* We were clearly meant to eat this planet's food, breathe its air, exercise and play on its land, swim in its waters, play with its animals, enjoy its sunlight, and live in harmony with its circadian rhythms.

One of the saddest statements I've ever heard is that people are digging their own graves with a fork, knife, and spoon. What makes it sad is that it's true. And worse, they are also digging that same grave with their sleep habits, their mental attitudes, and in other ways. This book will teach you how to use your fork, knife, and spoon, and other means at your disposal, to add zest and vitality to your life.

The very best of health to you!

David Klein
May, 2019

How to Use this Book

This book has been designed to improve your health and well-being by addressing most of the major health factors, dietary and otherwise. It's filled with an abundance of straightforward and logical points. So how should you approach the information in this book?

I recommend beginning by applying the points you believe will help you the most. And the more you apply them, the better you will do. But please, don't drive yourself crazy trying to master everything at once. Rather, enjoy the journey, the process. Give yourself credit when you make improvements. For instance, if you currently eat almost no healthy food, and you increase that amount to say 20 percent of your diet, you are headed in the right direction and are doing well. Find satisfaction in your progress, and rejoice with those smaller gains.

Mark key points in pen, highlighter, or on your reading device, and refer to them often as you are implementing them in your lifestyle.

You can read this book cover to cover if you like, or you can begin by reading the chapters that intrigue you the most, the ones that capture your interest.

And please, by all means, have fun. I had fun writing this volume, and I hope you have fun reading it and making health adjustments that lead to a happier, more vibrant life.

Dietary Enhancements

What we eat, how we eat, and when we eat have a huge impact on how we feel and on our well-being. Yet, there is a glaring confusion as to what constitutes a healthful diet. The world has made it a complicated matter, but it's really quite simple. This section will teach you how to eat for good and optimal health.

Is there a formula to stay trim, fit, and healthy? Yes, there is. It goes like this: *Eat the right foods, in the right amounts, at the right times. Give them a good chew too. And get moderate amounts of exercise.*

In this section, we'll focus on how you can make sure your diet provides you with optimal and vibrant health. Enjoy it.

What to Eat

1. "Eat the Rainbow"

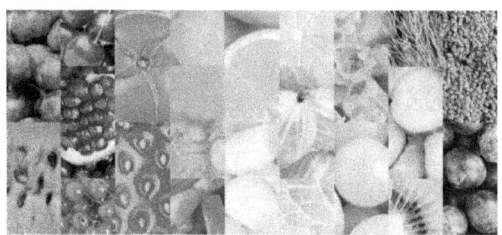

We'll start with one of the most important health tips: Eat the rainbow.

Eat the rainbow? That's an odd saying. But in modern health circles, it's a huge saying and it's packed with significance. What does it mean?

As we look in nature, we see there is an abundance of healthful, natural foods that grow out of the ground that are packed with vitamins, minerals, and enzymes. And those foods come in all colors and many shades of those colors. Hence, the term "eat the rainbow" refers to eating a wide variety of colorful natural foods. By doing this, you will likely be eating foods of all the colors in the rainbow. So when you are preparing your meals, be mindful of using a variety of colors. This is the foundation of a healthful diet, as it practically assures that you'll be getting the greatest amount of healthy nutrients from your food that you realistically can.

A sample rainbow of foods (the rainbow's colors are red, orange, yellow, green, blue, indigo, and violet):

Red: Cherries, Cranberries, Kidney Beans, Tomatoes, Strawberries, Watermelon

Orange: Apricot, Butternut Squash, Carrots, Mangoes, Oranges, Peaches, Pumpkin

4 Better Health: Happier Living

Yellow: Bananas, Chamomile, Corn, Grapefruit, Lemons, Yellow Squash

Green: Asparagus, Avocados, Celery, Cucumbers, Green Beans, Kale, Lettuce, Mint, Peas

Blue: Blueberries, Blue Corn

Indigo: Black Beans, Blackberries, Boysenberries, Plums, Prunes

Violet: Cabbage, Eggplant, Elderberries, Lavender, Passionfruit, Purple (Red) Onions

Each food color is reported to bring specific health benefits and nourish certain systems of the body. For instance, green foods, with their chlorophyll, are known to carry oxygen and to be cleansing, especially to the blood and liver; orange foods, with their beta carotene, build a strong immune system and fight diseases and cancer; red foods, with their anthocyanins and lycopene, protect heart health; and so forth. It's clear that eating a wide variety of natural foods brings many health benefits.

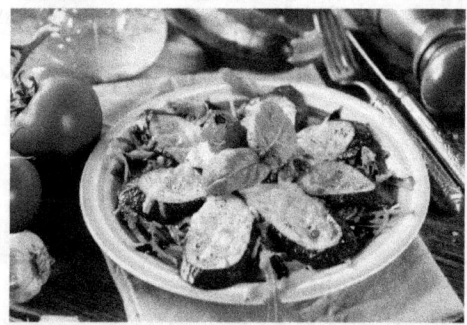

Note: The photos in this book appear in full color in Kindle editions. However, print editions of this book are produced in black and white. If you are reading a print edition, know that the photos of the rainbow of foods and the prepared dish are bursting with lively and nutritious colors. The photo of the junk foods? It doesn't look much different than it does in black and white. It's dull, and it's devoid of both color and nutrients.

Notice the picture of a conglomeration of junk foods. There's not much color, is there? The basic shade is dull brown; okay, a pale, lifeless, putrid dull brown. The human body was not meant to

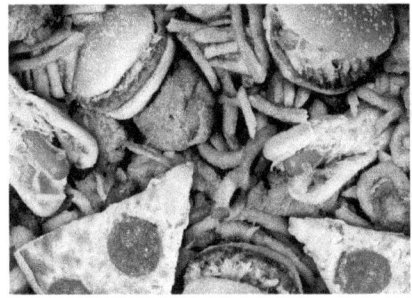

consume these foods, let alone to do so in large quantities as part of a steady diet. (I hesitated to use this picture in this book, because, let's face it, these foods are packed with carbs and fats and salt and can therefore taste good and be fun to eat. But when you look at this picture, think past your taste buds and view it from your body's point of view. Those foods are colorless because they are devoid of life-sustaining nutrients. What will eating a steady diet of these foods do to your body? Will they help it or will they hurt it?)

And speaking of good taste, you may be wondering if you can deal with trading in many of those colorless foods for the natural rainbow of foods. Will it be a boring venture? Will your diet become blasé?

No, it will not. Just as each natural food is decorated with a specific color, each is packed with a specific and delightful flavor. And here's the good part: The more you begin eating natural foods, and the less junk foods you eat, the more you'll enjoy those natural foods. The flavors will become more and more pronounced when your diet is clean, and you'll likely enjoy eating more than you did before. You'll get very excited about eating healthful, natural foods. (But don't expect this transformation to take place immediately. Usually, within a few weeks, you'll be enjoying your diet more than you previously did.) Keep at it. It's worth it.

2. Eat Natural Foods

Our Earth is a bespeckled jewel hanging in space, a wondrous treasured beauty. There is so much about it to love and enjoy. Near the top of that list for most of us is that it's a deep pantry of culinary delight. It's stocked with food, glorious food, occurring naturally in an abundance and an astounding variety, and that food is loaded with life-sustaining and health-building nutritional substances.

It may surprise you to know that there are an estimated 2,000 types of fruits and 20,000 types of vegetables. And those are just "types," not varieties.

For instance: An apple is one type of fruit, but there are 7,500 varieties of apples (Honeycrisp, Gala, Fuji, McIntosh, Pacific Rose, Red Royal Limbertwig, etc.) grown around the world today. That number is climbing, as new varieties are being grafted virtually every day. Each has a different taste and a different nutritional composition.

There is also a great variety of grains, nuts, seeds, legumes, and the list goes on. The number of spices alone is estimated by one source to be between 20,000 and 100,000. The Earth, indeed, is a well-stocked pantry of delightful edible treats. And those foods, in their natural states, have been proven to provide all of the healthful nutritious substances that we need to not only stay alive but to thrive.

As is often the case, though, man will try to find a better way to do things, often attempting to fix what is not broken. The main motives are convenience and, of course, profits.

Enter convenience foods. Cheese sprayed out of a can. Nutritious foods stripped of their sugar and the sugar being sold as a dangerous and ultimately lethal solo act. Oatmeal cut so finely that it becomes "quick cook," and in the process it becomes a "quick spike" to sugar and insulin levels. Wheat stripped of its nutrients and being sold, ton after ton, as white flour that resembles, and smells, like wallpaper paste.

Does that mean that the processing of foods is always harmful? Not at all. But for food to remain healthful, it should be minimally processed and only in accord with what is truly nourishing. As an example, is there anything wrong with processing the wonderful fruit olive into olive oil? Well, maybe. It depends on the processing method.

For instance, extra virgin olive oil, known also as EVOO, is truly a wondrous health food. Some of the healthiest people on the planet eat EVOO every day. You may wonder, though, what the term "extra virgin" refers to. Extra virgin olive oil is produced by crushing the olives to extract the liquid juice.

But now we get to the "maybe" part. Other grades of olive oils are produced differently. Chemicals are used to extract the juice from the olive. And those chemicals become part of the olive oil that is bottled and sold. So clearly, these other grades of olive oil are no longer truly natural, healthful foods, because they are chemically tainted.

If those lower grades of olive oil, or any oils, are subjected to the hydrogenation process, those oils become even less natural and way, way, more harmful. So again, processed foods are not necessarily to be avoided, but only when they are processed minimally and in harmony with non-destructive methods can they be considered truly natural or healthful.

Think of the huge variety of natural foods that grow out of the ground. There are literally thousands of them, perhaps even millions when all varieties are considered. Those foods are chock-full of a huge variety of nutrients that sustain our very lives. When your diet is made up primarily of a wide variety of healthful foods in their natural state, you will be rewarded with a bloom of health that you perhaps never thought possible.

3. Eat a Balance of Proteins, Fats, and Carbohydrates (The Three Macronutrients)

High protein, moderate protein, low protein, low carbohydrate, no carbohydrate, high complex carbohydrate, low fat, moderate fat, keto (fats coming out of your ears)—these are some of the health trends in just the last few decades. The three macronutrients are, for some reason, often at the center of a major dietary fad or trend.

What, though, is the truth regarding the macronutrients and a healthy diet?

Regarding proteins, fats, and carbohydrates, there are no villains. There are no superheroes either, as though one is better than the other. They are the three essential macronutrients, and they all play vital roles in building vibrant health. You need all three not only to function well, but to live. If the macronutrients are kept in reasonable balance and eaten in healthful forms, you can achieve better health.

So what is a proper balance of the three macronutrients? Of course, that can vary in individuals to some degree. However, since the principles of nutrition are sound and universal, the variance should not be a wild swing. Remembering that all three are vital to your health should help you keep your macronutrients in balance.

Some nutrition experts recommend that you achieve balanced meals in a way that is simpler and often more practical than counting grams of the various macronutrients. Here's how: You visually fill your plate with the proper proportions. They suggest filling half of your plate with non-starchy vegetables, such as salad, broccoli, asparagus, sautéed spinach, and so on; one-quarter of your plate with protein, such as fish, meat, or eggs; and one-quarter of your plate with healthy carbohydrates, such as a starchy vegetable, grain, or beans. What about fats? You should include some fats with each meal. Why? Fats slow down the absorption of carbohydrates and leave you feeling satisfied for a longer time after the meal. (So eating the proper amounts of fat at the proper times will not make you fat; quite the opposite: they will *prevent you* from becoming fat.) Some foods will supply proteins as well as fats, such as salmon or grass-fed beef. If your protein portion does not supply fat, you can add some olive oil or some nuts or seeds or perhaps half an avocado to boost fat content.

Finally, make sure to include all three macronutrients—proteins, carbohydrates, and fats—with each meal. Doing so will lead to a healthier, more balanced meal, better blood sugar control, a trimmer waistline, and enhanced enjoyment of your diet.

4. Eat Living Foods

Living foods refer to foods that still have life in them, such as enzymes. These include raw (uncooked) foods, sprouted foods, and cultured foods. The enzymes in living foods help your body in several ways.

Once foods are heated to a certain degree, the enzymes are damaged and can thus provide no benefit. Think of the difference between eating a raw food and eating the same food cooked: such as green peppers, carrots, or apples. While those foods are delicious when they are cooked and healthful to a degree, you can tell as you're chewing them that they are not living. There's no crunch, and the subtle taste of the raw flavors are no longer there. It's the same difference between drinking raw juices and eating soup. Soup is healthful, but if you really want to treat your body to a health boost, there's nothing like raw juice. It's alive, and it will give your body more life, more spark.

Some foods are better cooked, some even need to be cooked. For instance, I'm not about to dine on uncooked pinto beans or artichokes (ouch!). And while I have eaten raw potatoes, there's no question that I prefer them cooked. Don't be fanatical about living foods, feeling that you are breaking a law by eating cooked foods. Just be sure to eat a good amount of living foods in your daily diet. It adds zest to your health, and it makes a difference.

5. Drink Plenty of Water

Water. It's as simple as two parts hydrogen and one part oxygen. Yet, it's a miraculous, life-sustaining fluid. And we need lots of it to function and to function at our peak.

Make sure to drink enough high-quality water on a daily basis to meet your body's needs. The human body needs to stay well-hydrated to function at its best. How much water is enough? Of course, that depends on several factors, such as your body weight, your level of activity, the climate you live in, and so on. But there are some good rules of thumb that will work for most people.

One of these rules is to drink at least half of your body weight in ounces on a daily basis. So if you weigh 200 pounds, you should drink at least 100 ounces of water per day.

If you are like me and many others, you may find that it's difficult to drink that much water, especially out of a glass or cup. The solution? Drinking out of a water bottle, especially where you use a spout, or where your entire mouth can cover the drinking area, such as the type of bottle you buy in grocery stores in 24-packs, makes it much easier, and more enjoyable, to drink our daily water needs.

As a suggestion, it's best to drink the vast amount of your daily water during the day. Drinking too much water at night, and especially close to bedtime, will have a detrimental effect on your sleep. Running to the bathroom several times a night, and constantly interrupting and restarting your sleep cycles, is not restful.

Should you drink tap water? The answer is not so simple, and it depends upon several factors. One of those factors is your financial situation, as drinking copious amounts of bottled water can be expensive. Another factor is the quality of tap water where you live. Simply put, some municipalities supply better tap water than others. My take is this: For the most part, if you can afford it, you are better off drinking bottled or filtered water. A central theme in this book is to take control of your health and life, and you have zero control over what is added to your tap water. Where I live, the tap water wreaks of chlorine. ("A little bleach with your meal, sir?") Fluoride, chlorine, and other harmful substances are commonly added to tap water. Water may be the most important substance we consume, so it makes sense to ensure that the water we drink is as pure and healthful as possible.

Does lugging huge amounts of water to your home every time you go to the store seem like an unpleasant task? There's an option: You can install a reverse osmosis filtering system under your sink. Or, depending upon where you live, you can hire a service that not only installs the unit but that changes the filters for you periodically as needed.

Finally, listen to and obey your thirst. I may not be the most interesting man in the world, but I can offer this: Don't stay thirsty, my friends. That thirst signal is there for a reason . . . quench it.

6. Consider Eating Probiotics

This is one topic that is gaining increasing attention in recent years. And for good reason. So much of our well-being is determined by what is known as our "gut health." So what are probiotics, and how do they help us?

Probiotics are healthy bacteria. (*Pro* means "for" and *bio* means "life".) We need these bacteria in abundance in our digestive systems. There are an estimated (have fun trying to do an exact count!) 100 trillion microorganisms, from 500 unique species, in the normal healthy human bowel. Most of these are healthful, and they keep harmful microorganisms, known as "pathogens," from taking over and damaging our bodies.

Probiotics do a world of wonder for us: They not only fight pathogens, but they aid in digestion, nutrient absorption, and they boost immune function. In other words, you've got trillions of tiny friendly helpers working to make your life easier and your health better. Without these helpers you are more prone to several ailments of the digestive system, such as constipation, diarrhea, and urinary tract infections (UTIs), as well as other ailments, such as skin disorders.

Modern living and modern diet can severely reduce the amount of probiotics in the intestinal system. How can you boost your probiotic count? There are three basic ways:

a. Eat fermented foods that boost your probiotics.

The best sources of probiotic foods are foods that have been fermented. Fermented dairy products include yogurt, kefir, and buttermilk. Other fermented foods high in probiotics are non-dairy yogurts, such as those made from soy and coconut milk, sourdough bread, kimchi, sauerkraut, pickled vegetables, and kombucha. Currently, several of our close friends are making their own kombucha, and they enjoy the process thoroughly.

Note: When buying sauerkraut and pickled vegetables, make sure to buy only the types that need to be refrigerated, such as Bubbie's brand. The sauerkraut and pickles that you buy on the non-refrigerated aisles of the grocery store may taste good, but they are not sources of probiotics.

b. Take probiotic supplements.

Taking probiotic supplements can also add to the count of friendly bacteria in your body. Look for probiotics that are sold refrigerated, and continue to refrigerate your probiotics when you bring them home. Remarkably, the count of supplemental probiotics is often over 25 billion per capsule.

c. Take antibiotics only when necessary.

If *pro*biotics help the body, you can only imagine what *anti*biotics do. Antibiotics are often viewed as a wonder drug. The problem is, when you have finished your round, you're body wonders what just happened to it. And it's not pretty. While antibiotics may be necessary to wipe out a bacterial strain that your body is having trouble fighting off by itself, those antibiotics are also wiping out your healthy bacteria, the ones that work wonders in your digestive system and that are necessary for good health. Please use antibiotics only when they are medically necessary and there are no other viable options.

7. Consider Some Organic Foods

When I first heard about organic foods, I was perhaps in middle school in the late 1960s. The concept seemed odd to me. After all, what was wrong with the regular foods we'd been eating?

To my parents and especially grandparents, the concept of organic foods would have been really odd. Not too long ago, foods were grown on family-run farms in mostly organic fashion. But beginning perhaps in the early-to-mid 1900s, and escalating ever since, farming techniques have relied on chemicals to make crops more pest-resistant and more profitable. Profitable, in this case, means larger, heavier, altered produce.

However, there has been a weighty price to pay for such tampering. The foods retain some of the chemicals, lose much of their nutritional value, and in other ways they are poor imitations of the original, natural foods.

Try the banana test! The value of organic foods really hit home with me not too long ago with bananas. Simply put, I realized that as a child I liked bananas. They were not my favorite fruit, but they were still pretty high up there on the list. And yet, through the years, I noticed I had eaten less and less bananas until, in recent years, I stopped eating them completely. I never gave this much thought until my wife mentioned how bananas have changed: they didn't taste like they used to. She too had stopped eating bananas, referring to them as overly large, rubbery, and chemically tasting. That was exactly how I'd describe them too.

About this time my wife bought a few organic bananas. I tried one and could not believe what I was tasting. The banana was soft, and it actually tasted like . . . a banana, which was a flavor I had almost forgotten about through the years. This proved to be no fluke, as we've been eating organic bananas since, and every one has that soft, mellow, unique banana flavor we loved so much as children. Some (if not most) organic foods are worth the extra money if you can afford them. I'll never eat another bloated "rubber-chemical banana" again.

What Not To Eat

8. Don't Eat Refined Carbohydrates

We'll start off this section with a biggie. Refined carbohydrates are one of the most health-damaging things you can eat—and yet, they are everywhere. We're talking white sugar, white flour, high-fructose corn syrup, and so on. Refined carbohydrates are food fragments; wholesome foods have been stripped of their carbohydrates, and only the pure carbohydrate portion is sold. If you want to enjoy better health, you must eat very few refined carbohydrates. And if you want to enjoy excellent health, avoid them like the health plague that they've become.

Why are refined carbohydrate so damaging to our health? Notice this list, from a *Reader's Digest* article written by superb health writer Tina Donvito, titled "11 Scary Things Sugar Does to Your Body:" (Note: all refined carbohydrates have a very similar effect on the body as sugar; they all are rapidly converted to glucose.)

1. Sugar May Shorten Lifespan
2. Sugar Spikes Your Insulin
3. Sugar Puts You at Risk for Diabetes
4. Sugar Makes You Gain Weight
5. Sugar Ups Your Blood Pressure and Heart Disease Risk
6. Sugar Messes With Your Brain's Signals
7. Sugar Can Leave You Still Hungry
8. Sugar Makes Your Brain Suffer
9. Sugar Can Lead to Fatty Liver Disease
10. Sugar Can Rot Your Teeth
11. Sugar Raises Your Risk of Depression

That is some comprehensive list. And yet, there are people out there, literally millions of them, who are suffering with all 11 health plagues concurrently. Yes, all 11 at once. And they can't feel good or be truly content while their bodies and minds are being thus ravaged. How sad.

Please, consider eating refined carbohydrates to be your dietary enemy number one. And know that as soon as you stop eating them, all 11 items on that list will begin to improve for you, perhaps even drastically: You lose weight, your blood sugar stabilizes, your insulin levels drop—you look better, you feel better, and your risk of disease goes way down. That's quite a huge payoff for making just one change.

I'm by no means a fan of the keto diet. Nutritionally, it's a disaster, as it violates many, many known and accepted health rules. ("A little lard with your chemically saturated bacon, sir?") As I mention in my book *The Keto Diet Damaged our Health: A Better Approach*, in what rational world are bacon and lard considered health foods and carrots are not?

But, no doubt, people can and do lose weight on the keto diet. Why? It's not what they are eating that makes them lose weight, it's what they are not eating. And what is that? They've cut out all refined carbohydrates. In any diet, that's perhaps the number one way to lose weight. Most nutritionists don't like the keto diet because, as good as it is to cut out refined carbs, there are better ways to fill in the gaps than eating high amounts of fat. How much better to increase consumption of protein and of health-building, vitamin-and-mineral-chocked vegetables!

By the way, I would add one more effect of sugar, and all refined carbs, to Ms. Donvito's list. Sugar raises levels of the blood fat "triglycerides." High triglycerides are another risk factor for heart attack and stroke. You may wonder if the process of raised triglycerides is a slow, long-term matter. No, it's not. One of the main reasons you are directed to fast before taking a blood test is that carbohydrates, and especially refined carbohydrates, will raise your blood triglyceride level almost instantly and thus alter your report.

Some well-intentioned people who want to break free from refined carbohydrates will substitute with a like amount of natural sugars, such as fruit. Doing so is an improvement, but still not the answer, as excessive sugars, even ones in their natural form, still carry some of the same health risks, but to a lesser degree.

Is there a viable solution? Yes, you can use a healthful form of a sugar substitute. I'd recommend one, or a combination, of the following three: Stevia, Lo Han (Monk Fruit Extract), and Xylitol. All are natural, and all are essentially carb and glycemic free. Try them all, and perhaps various brands of each, to see if you have a favorite. In our household, we use a combination of all three: stevia, monk fruit, and xylitol. You can also add to that mix, *in small amounts*, such natural sugars as honey and pure maple syrup.

You may wonder what types of carbohydrates are healthful to eat. Basically, all carbohydrates in their natural state, which means *unrefined*, are healthful. These include vegetables, fruits, grains, beans, and many other sources. Since some carbohydrate foods have a higher amount of simples sugars and total sugar content, such as many fruits, exercise care not to eat too many carbohydrates, even natural ones, and especially don't eat too many at one time, which will spike your blood sugar level.

By eating natural carbohydrates in moderation, avoiding refined carbohydrates, and using healthful sugar substitutes, you will be on your way to reaching your health and weight goals.

9. Don't Eat Bad Fats

Many, many years ago, I was out with some friends who wanted to go to a popular fast food restaurant for a quick lunch. A young engaged couple was with our group, and I could not help but notice the beauty of the bride-to-be. In fact, she closely resembled a famous actress who was also a supermodel at the time.

This young lady had ordered French fries, and the discussion of how unhealthy fries are to the body was raised. I wanted to make a point about how much oil was in French fries, so I asked if I could have one, and then I put it in a napkin and squeezed. It was not pretty. A good portion of the napkin was saturated in oil, and it looked more like grease or car lubricant than it did food. (In case you are wondering, oh yes, the young lady was none too pleased with me—but she was very gracious about it.)

That was clearly a case of bad fat: greasy, deep fried, colorless, thick sludge on a napkin. But if that were, say, fresh extra virgin olive oil, the appearance on the napkin would not be greasy and there would be a pleasing golden-green color to the oil.

Fats are a necessary part of the human diet. But just as there are good carbs and bad carbs, there are also good fats and bad fats.

So what are good fats and what are bad fats? Like so many other food matters described in this book, good fats are the ones that occur naturally and are minimally processed; bad fats are ones that have been altered in such a way as to make them unhealthful or even carcinogenic.

Some of the best examples of good fats are nuts, seeds, and avocados. Oils can fall into the category of good fats or bad fats. Anything deep fried is a bad fat. Some oils, such as canola oil, are currently a source of debate; some nutritionists recommend canola oil, and others do not. The safest and most universally accepted oil is olive oil, especially in the form of "extra virgin," which is often designated by the initials EVOO. Avocado oil is considered healthy, as are a few other oils.

Keep in mind that oils are very concentrated sources of calories. Fat contains more than double the calories of the same amount of protein or carbohydrates. So eat healthy fats, but eat them in moderation.

If at all possible, never, ever eat deep fried foods. They are a health hazard in so many ways. They cause an increase in risk of heart attack, stroke, and cancer, and your poor stomach has no idea what to do with the grease. In teens, especially, the grease will form eruptions (pimples) on the skin. It will make you look bloated, fat, off-color and just not good.

Another must-to-avoid are trans fats. Trans fats are oils that have been partially hydrogenated, which makes them semi-solid and more stable at room temperature. They are used commonly in margarines, packaged baked goods, potato chips, and other similar foods. Trans fats are a health hazard. Some countries even impose legal limits on the amount of trans fats allowed in foods sold.

What about saturated fats, which have so often been misunderstood. Saturated fats are generally less healthy than unsaturated fats. Yet, they occur naturally in many foods and are fine in small amounts.

So remember, fats are neither to be glorified as a superfood—keto, or avoided practically like the plague—Pritikin. (That said, some with serious health disorders, such as heart disease, may be encouraged by their physician to adhere to a diet that is very low in fat.) Rather, fats are an essential part of any good diet . . . but only in moderation, and only the good fats, not the bad ones.

10. Don't Eat Chemicals

I love this chapter heading. It's probably the most "duh" heading in this book. We are supposed to eat food, not chemicals. And yet, we eat tons of them. Some of them are fairly harmless in small doses; others are, simply put, poison to the body.

This is one subject that most of the population really doesn't understand, but the impacts of chemicals in our diets is huge. (What's to understand about names like "Glucono delta-lactone" and "Sodium carboxymethyl cellulose"?) Our foods are flooded with all types of man-made chemicals and some grotesque natural substances—the manufacturers do this for a bunch of small reasons but really for one main reason.

Some of the small reasons our foods are chemically drenched: to keep them fresher longer, to make them bigger and better looking, to make them more colorful, to keep them free of pests, to make them softer, to make them harder, to make them taste better, and so on. The main reason, sadly, has to do with greens—not the type that you eat, but the type that you deposit in a bank, or rather, the type that the manufacturers of these foods deposit in *their* banks. Profit rules big business, and sadly, it frequently does so at the cost of our health.

This is probably a good time to introduce the work of Vani Hari, otherwise known as the Food Babe. Vani has dedicated her working hours to exposing the harmful additives in commercial foods and then putting lots of pressure on the manufacturers to remove the offending items.

We probably all know that such foods as diet sodas are mostly chemicals and carbonated water (which makes diet sodas excellent car battery cleaners—try cleaning your car battery with carrot juice . . . I don't think you'll have much success, and please don't attempt this unless you drive an orange-colored vehicle.)

But note some other substances that are added to the foods you eat, as explained in the foreword to Vani Hari's best-selling book *The Food Babe Way*. Renowned doctor Mark Hyman, who wrote the foreword, points out: "Most of us are completely oblivious to what we are eating and its impact on our health and our world. We know little about how our food is grown; how our seeds are engineered; how our farming methods harm the soil, air, and water, and contribute to climate change and dead zones in our oceans. We are mostly unaware of the chemicals that are added to our foods and how the hormones, antibiotics, plastics, and toxins we eat in our everyday foods harm our bodies. How could we know that we are eating Silly Putty in our French fries and yoga mat softeners in our bread; or cancer-causing preservatives such as BHA and BHT, which have been banned in every country but ours, or that dyes and coloring agents in our macaroni and cheese may cause hyperactivity and behavioral problems in our children; or that natural flavors are made from ground up animal parts; or that common foods contain secretions from beavers' anal glands?"

That passage goes on, but mercifully, I'll stop there.

You may be surprised to learn that some food items, including restaurant foods, contain upwards of fifty or even one hundred ingredients. It's exhausting reading those lists, but it's more exhausting to the body to try to figure out what to do with those items, many of which are chemicals that have no business being in food in the first place.

The solution: eat simple and natural foods, especially ones that you prepare yourself. Don't trust that the food industry has your best interests at heart; it doesn't, because profits are a powerful motivating choice when determining what goes into the foods companies sell. Buck that trend, and take control of what you eat. It's your body, and it's one that you want to serve you well for as long as possible.

And a big thank you to Vani, the Food Babe, and others, for bringing these things to our attention and trying to protect our well-being.

11. Don't Eat Junk Food

You may be surprised at the brevity of this chapter, and there is a good reason for that, as follows: The three previous chapters, under the section "What Not to Eat," were entitled Don't Eat Refined Carbohydrates, Don't Eat Bad Fats, and Don't Eat Chemicals. Simply put, if you avoid eating refined carbs, bad fats, and chemicals, you almost automatically will be eliminating all junk foods from your diet, because those are the primary ingredients in junk foods. In other words, they are what make junk junk.

The saying *We Are What We Eat* is not really accurate. If it were, I don't think chopped liver would ever be on my menu. Yet, that saying has some merit, but perhaps it would be better written as: *What We Eat Will Have a Major Impact on Our Health*. Eating junk food will wreck our health, whereas eating healthful food will build our health. Vitamins, minerals, and enzymes will help us; aspartame, sucralose, BHT, BHA, MSG, high-fructose corn syrup, sugar, trans fat, and deep fried oils will harm us. (To add to the list of inedible acronyms, never eat GTOs. Even if they are served with a V-8, they are rough on digestion and a nightmare for your liver to process.)

The more wise health and dietary choices you make, the more you'll reap the benefits of those choices. Good health is a delightful gift, and it's one to be valued and guarded.

Experience: *Eating For Beauty: Natural Foods Versus Junk Foods.* When I was in my mid-20s, I had an experience that taught me the importance of diet and physical appearance . . . I was living in Southern California and had been on a very clean, rainbow-type oriented diet. My health improved dramatically. And then I discovered Mexican food, including fast Mexican food. I began to eat lots of it, and for a period of at least a few months I left my healthy diet behind, and I began to eat lots of the types of foods that you see in the "junk foods" picture we discussed in an earlier chapter. One night, a friend and I ate a meal at a local fast food Mexican restaurant, and when I returned home, I realized that I left my wallet at my seat in the restaurant. I immediately returned, asked about my wallet, and the staff denied having seen it.

So much for my wallet. For the next several days, I went through the process of replacing the contents of my wallet, including my driver's license, which required my taking another photograph at the DMV office.

About two months later, guess what showed up in the mail? That's right, someone had dropped my wallet, minus the cash in it, in a mailbox, and the postal service returned it to me. So now I had two driver's licenses, and I was shocked by how different I looked in the photos, one of which was taken while I was on a clean, rainbow-oriented diet, and the other while I was in the middle of my Mexican food binge period—remember, it was a Mexican fast food restaurant where I lost my wallet in the first place.

I never claimed to be a beauty, but in the first picture, my skin looked clean, my complexion was bright, my face was trim, and my eyes were clear. In the second photo, I looked like an entirely different person: my skin looked dark and blotchy, my face was bloated, and my eyes had no shine. Really, I looked like two different people, and those photos were taken only about a year or so apart. I knew right then it was time to clean up my diet again.

12. If You Have Food Allergies or Sensitivities, Avoid Those Foods

Have you heard about food allergies and sensitivities? Are you skeptical? There's no need to be. Food allergies and sensitivities are real, and they can wreak havoc on our bodies and our minds.

(Note: Food allergies and food sensitivities are similar, but each has a distinct effect on the body. Food allergies can be the most severe, and even one molecule of the offending substance can cause the body to react and go into immediate shock. Food sensitivities are more subtle, and they are sometimes referred to as "delayed food allergies," as the symptoms may not become manifest for several minutes, hours, or even a couple of days. Both food allergies and sensitivities involve and affect the immune system. For simplicity sake, I use both terms interchangeably in this chapter.)

Some food allergies are very obvious. For instance, a small group of people are allergic to peanuts, and the allergy is severe. Just one peanut, or even a pinhead size of peanut butter, can cause shock or even death. There was a news article a few years ago about a person who was allergic to shellfish, who was dining at a restaurant, when a food server merely walked by his table with a plate of steaming shellfish. Inhaling the steam alone caused that person to go into shock and die.

Most food allergies and sensitivities are less severe and less noticeable, and they create less of a problem, but they can still do a number on us, especially over time. Common allergens are wheat, dairy, eggs, peanuts, shellfish, gluten, and many others.

How do you know if you have a food allergy? There are many methods of testing for food allergies. But even without testing, there are often clear signs that would indicate an allergy to a certain food. One sign is very obvious: You likely are allergic to a food if, after eating it, you consistently develop a specific physical symptom. So if you break out in a rash every time you eat, say, products with corn, you are almost surely allergic to corn. My easiest allergy to detect is aged cheese. If I eat some parmesan, feta, or other aged cheese, my skin will begin to itch almost immediately. Then when I wake up the next day, my IQ seems to drop in half, as my brain feels like it's wrapped in a thick fog. It's no fun, and I avoid aged cheese at virtually all costs. (I desperately miss those 20 IQ points when that happens.)

But there is another sign of being allergic to a food that is a little trickier—actually, it's a lot trickier: If there is a food that you are repeatedly drawn back to, because you love eating it and it immediately makes you feel better, such as more energized, you likely are allergic to that food. Keep in mind that we all have food preferences. We simply like certain foods more than others, and that's normal. But if our pull to a certain food is unusually strong, to where that food is almost a must for us each day and perhaps each meal, we may be allergic to it. But why is that so? Why would we be drawn to a food we are allergic to?

The answer is "adrenal hits". When we eat the offending food, our body reacts to it. But the reaction to this food is not so noticeable and it actually feels good, not bad. No rash, no headache, no itching, etc. Our body reacts by trying to neutralize the damage from the food, so it releases extra cortisol and adrenaline. That provides a "rush" to our system, and it seems to give us more energy, which feels good. But as with a sugar "rush," in a short while we are weaker than we were before the rush. How can we feel better again? Only one way: eat more of that same food for another rush. And the cycle has begun: Eat the offending food, get an energy rush, come down from that rush to a lower level, eat the offending food again, another rush, and so on.

If you remember my aged-cheese allergy: I have no desire to eat aged cheese at all. But I also have a strong chocolate allergy. Do I have a desire to eat chocolate? There are three answers to that question: Yes, YES, and, **YES**. Okay, there is a fourth answer: **YES!** If I could, I'd eat chocolate all day every day. Semi-dark 50% cocoa will do just fine, thank you. In fact, once I begin eating chocolate, it's extremely difficult to stop. And I want my next meal to be . . . more chocolate, not to mention several chocolate snacks in between. My allergy/addiction is so strong that I have decided to forego eating chocolate at all. Just one bite and my health suffers from the inevitable roller coaster addiction again.

If you learn what foods you're allergic to, and you avoid them, your body will be spared from the constant ups and downs of the adrenal hits caused by those foods and eventual adrenal exhaustion. If you don't avoid them completely, please know that the more you do avoid them, the less stress there will be on your body.

True Story: You may have caught it, or you may not have, but I placed the fourth "**YES!**", the large one, in a dark brown font to replicate the color of chocolate. (This will be evident in Kindle editions of this book but not paperback copies, which are printed in black and white.) Just to show you how strong a food allergy/addiction can be, a day or so after changing the color of the font, when I went back to add to this section, I noticed that font, and I actually began to instantly crave dark chocolate—just from the color alone. The point: food allergies are real, and if you crave a certain food inordinately, you likely are allergic to it. Even though it makes you feel better when you first eat it, that allergy could be undermining your health and well-being. It may be good to be checked for food allergies if you have this dilemma.

When to Eat

13. Don't Skip Breakfast, and Make it a High-Protein Meal

One of the best recent trends among nutritionists is to recommend that we eat high-protein breakfasts. It makes a lot of sense. Breakfasts have increasingly become a carbohydrate-fest. Throw that quick energy down the gullet and buzz out the door. It feels pretty good at the time, but in about an hour or two you have stopped buzzing and it doesn't feel so good anymore. The stage is actually set for a day of dietary misery and weight gain.

Dietary misery and weight gain? Yes. A high-carbohydrate breakfast, such as dry cereal with milk and sugar, a Danish, and a glass of orange juice, will provide an immediate and substantial spike in blood sugar. Such a meal has a drug addiction-like effect on the body, as sugar-lowering insulin is released and the quick high is followed by a quick low. And there's only one way to fix that quick low . . . get another quick high. How? Another high-carb snack or meal. If you eat a high-carb breakfast, the roller coaster effect of high and low sugar will begin for the day. That's exhausting to the body, and it packs on the pounds.

A high-protein breakfast sets the stage for a day of balanced meals. Protein doesn't provide the spike in sugar that carbohydrates do—the protein meal sustains you much longer—so you'll be much less prone to cravings for sweets during the day.

A high-protein breakfast does not mean an ALL-protein breakfast. It's good to include small-to-moderate amounts of carbohydrates and fat. So what constitutes a good breakfast? Aim for at least 20-25 grams of protein, and limit the fat content to perhaps 10-15 grams and the carbohydrate amount to 15-25 grams, or perhaps higher if you are very physically active. So a breakfast of 2-3 eggs or 4-6 ounces of animal protein, a *small* serving of cooked natural-grain cereal, with a little olive oil or butter on the cereal, and a small piece of fruit (perhaps a few slices of an apple, a few slices of a not-too-ripe banana, or some berries) may be about ideal.

Keep in mind that you don't have to have your breakfast the moment you get out of bed. But if you need a quick pick up, you can start your day with a handful of nuts or seeds or a small piece of fruit. Then, maybe thirty to sixty minutes later, you can have your full breakfast. Listen to your body and see what works best for you.

Some people simply don't have much of an appetite in the morning, and others don't have the time or inclination to prepare a meal when they first wake up. A good solution: My favorite nutritional expert, Dr. Alan Christianson, who I refer to often in this book, recommends a protein shake for breakfast. Personally, I've found this to be the ideal breakfast. I'll use a base of perhaps unsweetened almond, flax, or coconut milk, or a combo of them, add in about 25 grams of a good protein powder, add a helping of sunflower seeds, chia seeds or flax seeds, then maybe a teaspoon of honey, and finally some non-glycemic sweetener, such as monk fruit, stevia, or xylitol. You can also add some fruit or vegetables to your shake. If you add some toasted carob powder, you might just think you are eating a chocolate shake for breakfast.

Adding some resistant starch to your shake makes the energy boost of your breakfast shake last even longer. Resistant starch is, as the name implies, resistant to something . . . and that something is digestion. Therefore, resistant starch digests more slowly and provides energy for a longer period of time. Good sources of resistant starch are bananas with some green on them, green banana flour, and white beans, such as navy beans, great northern beans, and cannellini beans. Don't discard the beans' liquid, called aquafaba, which is also very high in resistant starch.

The morning protein shake is quick, it's nutritious, it's tasty, and it's an excellent dietary start to the day.

14. Don't Eat More Than a Snack Late in the Evening

Your diet and your sleep are intertwined. Have a bad night's sleep, or hardly get any sleep, and for most people that's the perfect storm to eat the wrong foods and to eat too much of them the following day.

What's one of the surest ways to get a bad night's sleep? Eat a large meal late in the evening. Why is this so? The body and the brain both need and crave quality sleep, but they are only able to get quality sleep when they can truly rest. Digesting a meal is a huge task for both the body and brain. How so? The body spends much energy in digesting and assimilating food. Virtually all of the major organs are involved and at work; digestion is like a symphony between many organs. And the brain? It's the conductor of that symphony, and it must be alert, neurons firing away, to direct everything that's going on.

The body needs to do a few things while asleep, and that's essentially to rest, to heal, to cleanse, and to renew. The brain needs to do gazillions of things, including rest, process the day's events, and dream about any myriad of things. If your brain is busy with the digestive process, it won't get the rest it needs, and it won't be able to benefit from the mentally and emotionally restorative process of dreaming.

Finally, it's a proven fact that both laboratory animals and humans eat more when they are deprived of the necessary quantity and quality of sleep. So by eating a meal late at night, we initiate a dangerous cycle: Poor night's sleep, fatigue during the day, overeating, including late at night, another poor night's sleep, and so on. Break that cycle by, as a general practice, refraining from eating more than a snack past, perhaps, 7:00 pm or thereabouts. You don't have to go to bed hungry, you can have a snack, but keep it light and chew it well.

15. Cycle Your Carbohydrates

Carbohydrate cycling refers to the practice of starting the day with a high-protein, low-carbohydrate meal, and then increasing carbohydrate intake as the day progresses. It's not only *what* you eat that is important, but also *when* you eat.

Carbohydrate cycling works in harmony with the body's natural rhythms, as carbohydrates are not as necessary early in the day when the cortisol levels are at their peak and the body has lots of stored energy from a good night's sleep. Carbohydrate intake becomes more important as the day goes on and the cortisol levels slope downward. Further, eating too many carbohydrates early in the day starts the process of blood sugar highs and resulting lows for the entire day. A higher protein breakfast gets your day off to a smoother start, and it prevents those sugar spikes and the ensuing carbohydrate cravings.

Does carbohydrate cycling mean bacon and eggs for breakfast, a sandwich and apple for lunch, and pasta washed down with a Big Gulp for dinner? Not at all. With carbohydrate cycling, the rules of healthy nutrition must be followed.

All three meals must include a good mix of healthy proteins, fats, and carbohydrates. The protein and fat content will remain similar for all three meals, but the carbohydrate content would be low at breakfast, higher at lunch, and even higher (though never too high) at dinner. The carbohydrate portion should consist of healthy whole grains; starchy vegetables, such as yams, sweet potatoes, potatoes, and carrots; beans, and fruits. As a rule, most people would do well to limit carbohydrate intake to about 100 grams per day. So, as an example, you may want to have about 15 grams of carbohydrates at breakfast, about 30 at lunch, and about 40 at dinner, with the remaining 15 grams spread among daily snacks.

You may want to give carbohydrate cycling a try to see if it works for you.

How to Eat

16. Chew Your Food Thoroughly

This is an often overlooked health topic, but chewing thoroughly provides a *huge* boost to your level of health.

Chewing your food thoroughly brings many benefits. First, it slows down your meal, and that alone brings two main benefits. 1. It slows the release of sugar into your system. When your sugar level spikes quickly, that will be followed by a corresponding rapid insulin spike, which will lower your blood sugar. That's a guarantee of one thing: that you will soon crave a quick carb fix to get your sugar back up. That one rushed meal will begin an unwanted sugar high-low cycle for the entire day or longer. 2. Your brain has a built in hunger-stopping mechanism. When you've eaten enough food, the brain sends a signal that it's time to stop eating. But that satiation signal has a little built-in time delay. If you eat too quickly, you'll have eaten several bites before the signal has time to take effect. That leads to overeating, which, for your health, is never a good thing.

Chewing thoroughly brings other important benefits. Digesting food is quite a workload for your body. True, it's an involuntary action, but that does not mean it's a simple or easy task for the body, which it is not. Where does the digestive system begin? In the mouth. The rest of the digestive system is literally at the mercy of the mouth, because only the mouth has a voluntary role in digestion. Once the food gets past the mouth, it's all involuntary from there. But when you make the decision to chew your food thoroughly, you are aiding the digestive process in two ways:

First, and probably foremost, chewing to break food down into small particles is absolutely vital to good digestion. Your teeth are designed to chew food; your stomach is not. If you were to forego chewing, the rest of the digestive system would have its workload multiplied exponentially. And still, it could not do as thorough a job as it could if the food were well chewed. (This creates a huge energy drain on your body's resources. Would you rather spend your energy in play, in getting essential work done, in spending time with your friends and family, or would you rather spend it digesting food that you've neglected to chew?)

Second, saliva is loaded with substances that start the process of digestion right in the mouth. By breaking your food down with your teeth and saturating it with saliva, your digestive process gets a huge head start and has a much easier workload.

As an example, think, if you will, about eating a handful of cashews. Cashews are dry, solid, and have a definite shape. But when you chew them, they quickly turn into a moist smooth paste. That's very easy work for your mouth. Picture both scenarios now: either those dry, hard, whole cashews reaching your stomach, or the smooth and liquefied cashew paste you've made with your mouth doing so. I'm sure you can see the difference from your stomach's point of view. What in the world will it do with those whole cashews, or even cashew pieces for that matter? It doesn't have teeth and can't do the job. That food will remain largely undigested and a burden to the system.

To further illustrate the benefits of thorough chewing, you might want to try this: Get a nice, juicy, sweet apple. Either take a bite of the apple or cut a slice and put it in your mouth. Then begin to chew the apple as you focus on the taste sensation in your mouth. Don't swallow any of the pulp; just chew on the apple pieces and pay attention to the juice being separated from the pulp. Swallow only the juice as you are chewing. When the juice has been completely extracted and swallowed, then you may swallow the pulp.

What will you find? If the apple is a high quality apple with good texture, taste, and sweetness, you'll notice how quickly the juice is extracted from the pulp when you chew. And that juice is sweet, delightful, and the freshest juice you'll ever taste. And when you've finished each "sip" of the juice (each mouthful), you'll chase that down with the fibrous pulp, which brings additional health benefits.

Your taste buds, your brain, your digestive system, and your entire body get a delightful treat.

But now think about what happens if you merely chew that piece of apple only a few times, just enough to break it up so the pieces are small enough to swallow. The juice is not extracted from the pulp, and those pieces end up in your stomach in a wet, acidic environment, sitting there for hours at 98.6 degrees Fahrenheit (37 degrees Celsius) before they can be inefficiently digested. Do you think you'll be getting any benefits of fresh raw juice that way?

There's an old saying: "Drink your solids and chew your liquids." That's excellent advice. Give your body a break by chewing your foods thoroughly. Your body will thank you . . . not verbally, of course, but with extra energy, more vibrant health, better digestion, and in many other ways.

17. Don't Overeat

Eating, needless to say, is very good for our health. Overeating is very bad for our health. Sadly, many people formed an overeating habit early in life, often at the encouragement of their parents to 'clean their plate.' Instead of eating to satisfaction, they eat until they are full . . . okay, stuffed. And they do this pretty much at every meal, and even all day long. What are the results?

Go to your local Walmart or wherever else the general public gathers and look around. Obesity is an epidemic, and it's not getting better. Some people, in a mere thirty or forty years of life, are so large that they can't even walk, and if they can, it's with great difficulty. Usually, when they get to that point, there's almost no turning back. (But it can be done by some who possess great motivation and moxie.)

Notice please some of the problems caused by frequent overeating:

- Obesity
- Heart Disease
- Diabetes
- High Cholesterol
- High Blood Pressure
- Stroke
- Cancer
- Excessive Doctor's Visits
- Digestive Disorders
- Social Issues and Low Self-Esteem
- Lower-Body Joint Pain
- Heartburn
- Exhaustion
- Back and Spine Problems
- Sleep Apnea
- Knee Problems
- Financial Problems, Including Frequent Wardrobe Adjustments
- Lack of Physical Conditioning
- Loss of Mobility
- Mood Swings
- Guilt
- Preoccupation with Body Weight
- Early Death

Stop the trend now. Remember, gaining only one pound per month will get you in trouble fast. That's 12 pounds a year, 48 pounds in four years, 120 pounds in ten years, 240 pounds in twenty years, 360 pounds in thirty years, and 480 pounds in 40 years.

One of the best ways to avoid overeating is to eat slowly and chew well. That extends your time with a meal, providing more enjoyment with less food, and it allows the hunger stop-signal to kick in before you've downed another 200 unnecessary calories. Working with the body's signals and rhythms is to your benefit. Overeating, clearly is not.

There's two more related problems with overeating: 1. If you have food sensitivities and allergies, which almost everyone does, you'll be subjecting your body to more of the foods that cause distress to your system. In fact, chances are good that the foods you overeat are the ones that you are sensitive or allergic to. 2. It's a sad fact that foods today, unless they are organic, are laden with chemicals that are not fit for human consumption. Eating more of those foods than is necessary will increase the chemical load on your body.

The solution: eat healthy foods and moderate amounts of those foods. Keep your diet clean and lean. It makes a huge difference to your health and life.

18. How Much Should You Eat?

Eating the proper amount of food is very important. On the one hand, you don't want to eat so little that you are weak, undernourished, or malnourished. On the other hand, you don't want to eat so much that you continually gain weight and suffer with the perils of being overweight or obese.

There are basically two ways to gage this matter. One is by the scale. If you remain close to your ideal body weight, and especially if you are trim at the waist, you are probably eating the right amount of food. (See Waist-Height Chart on page 75.) If you are overweight and are slowly but consistently losing weight, you are probably also eating the right amount of food for your circumstances. If you are gaining weight and continue to do so, even at the rate of a few pounds a year, you are eating too much food and need to make an adjustment. Gaining six pounds a year (which is only two ounces each week) equals some pretty serious obesity in a mere ten or twenty years.

The other way, the built-in way, is to go by your hunger. The hunger signal is a gift that allows you to know when to begin eating and when to stop. It's very reliable, unless it has been ignored or abused for a long period of time. But even in that case, the hunger signal can make a big-time comeback when you begin to pay attention to it and treat it with respect.

A wonderful graphic, called the Food Hunger Chart, has been developed. It lists the ten stages of hunger, and it's exceptionally helpful to visualize when you should begin eating a meal and when you should stop eating that meal.

Food Hunger Chart

- 1—Starving, weak, dizzy
- 2—Very hungry, cranky, low energy, lots of stomach growling
- 3—Pretty hungry, stomach is growling a little
- 4—Starting to feel a little hungry
- 5—Satisfied, neither hungry nor full
- 6—A little full, pleasantly full
- 7—A little uncomfortable
- 8—Feeling stuffed
- 9—Very uncomfortable, stomach hurts
- 10—So full you feel sick

So how do you navigate the Food Hunger Chart to your advantage? Notice these guidelines below:

Begin to eat when you are at level 3 or 4. If you reach level 2, you'll likely be so ravenous that you'll make poor food choices, wolf down your food, chew insufficiently, and overeat.

Stop eating at level 5 or 6. It's not on the chart, but if you want to imply a level of 5 ½, that may be close to an ideal level to stop eating.

Try to remain between levels 3 and 6 at all times. Those are your natural, healthy levels.

Recognize that it is normal and healthy to feel a little hungry in between meals. (Levels 3 and 4.) This is a sign that you are not overeating, and that's a good thing.

When you are trying to lose weight, don't allow yourself to go as low as levels 1 or 2. (Big mistake!) Rather, try to spend all of your time at levels 3, 4 and 5, with more time in level 4 than usual. Level 4 is the ideal weight loss level, but you want to bump up to level 5 two or three times a day to keep your energy up, to keep you going, and to keep you sane.

Eat slowly. There's a little delay of a few minutes in the satiation signal. If you eat too quickly, you might run past level 5 or 6 to level 7 before you know it.

Consider eating multiple smaller meals, perhaps five or six, per day. By doing this, you will have less swing in your movement between levels.

Eating balanced meals, containing a healthful mixture of proteins, carbs, and fats, will help you to recognize when you have eaten enough. And when you have, stop. It won't be long until it's time for your next snack or meal; having that to look forward to should help you to move on to another activity.

19. Keep Plenty of Healthful Foods on Hand; Keep Junk Foods out of the Home if Possible

You know the routine . . . it's mid-afternoon, you get hungry, and you decide to eat something healthful as your snack. Perhaps a nice small salad with lettuce, onions, carrots, tomatoes, and avocados, topped with a little canned tuna. You open the fridge, and the only lettuce you see is a wilted head of iceberg, clearly past its prime. You have one-half onion, but no carrots or tomatoes, and you have two avocados . . . one is as hard as a baseball and the other clearly passed the guacamole stage two weeks earlier. There's no tuna in the pantry either. But while you are in the refrigerator you notice a piece of your favorite pie or cake. What's going to happen next? For most of us, we know the answer to that.

It's often overlooked, but a key to dietary success is to have the right foods on hand. Having them prepared in advance, if possible, is even better. We are trying to balance three factors: 1. We want to eat more nutritious foods and to be healthier. 2. We want our food to taste good. 3. We are busy people, and realistically, convenience is usually going to win. You can stack the odds of success in your favor by having healthful, tasty, nutritious foods in the home and as ready to eat as possible.

The same principle applies when you are away from home. Having a bag of seeds, nuts, some fruit, raw vegies, or something else you like will get you out of many jams and keep your diet on track.

20. If You Fall Off the Dietary Bandwagon, Get Right Back On

It's the rare person who does not "cheat" on a diet. But those who are successful know how to "cheat" and then immediately get back on track. A reasonable cheat here and there won't submarine your health, but remaining in the dietary gutter will.

At times you may want to plan in advance to cheat. Suppose you are attending a wedding or some other gala event. Have a plan ahead of the occasion. Know how far off your diet you are willing to go for the occasion, and then be determined to get right back on it the next day. Such planning keeps you in control, and it can save lots of dietary blowouts, crashes, and heartaches.

21. Is Fasting Really Healthy? An Alternative.

Fasting was a huge trend circa the 1980s. It would have been even a bigger trend except for one "minor" detail about fasting: fasting involves not eating. Some people don't like not eating.

But concerning health benefits, books about fasting were being published at breakneck speed, and many if not most holistic doctors were on the fasting bandwagon, recommending it to their patients.

Did the fast fad last? No, and for good reason. An unexpected problem became evident, and many who fasted were disappointed with the results.

Most people, of course, lost weight during their actual fast period. But shortly after they had completed the fast, many gained more weight back than they lost. Those people were sure that they were being careful as to what and how much they ate, so it was puzzling as to why they were gaining weight.

Here's what researchers concluded: The body, in its wisdom, viewed the fast as an emergency, as a period of food scarcity. (The body doesn't know if your fast is intentional or not. For all it knows, you are lost in the woods and haven't had access to food for several days.) So the body would go into conservation mode, where it would hold onto as much weight as possible. Again, during the fast, you are still going to lose weight, even in this mode, because of the lack of food. But when you have decided that your fast is over, your body doesn't flip a switch and join you. It remains in conservation mode, and you actually gain more weight with the same amount of food as you were previously eating. Repeated fasts make this weight-gaining conservation mode stronger. So fasting was, in the long run, causing people to gain weight rather than lose weight.

And here's another problem with fasting: people were losing lots of lean muscle mass during their fasts. Because fasting, even juice fasting, is so lacking in protein, the body would begin to burn muscle as fuel.

So you may wonder, are there any alternatives to fasting? Yes, there are, and I'll discuss two here. The first one is my own creation, and the second is one created by a fabulous nutritional doctor, one whose praises I sing in this book several times.

The first is to eat, for a period of time of your choice, such as 3 days, 7 days, 10 days, 14 days, etc., only healthful foods, or at least as high a percentage of healthful foods as possible. Reduce the amount of food you eat; eat only as much food as you need to reasonably sustain yourself and to keep going with your life. Finally, chew your food very, very well, making, essentially, your solids into liquid before you swallow each bite. By doing this, you are significantly easing the load on your digestive system, your heart, and so on. You're getting mostly all the nutrients you need, but the load on your system is minimal because the foods are healthful, there's not an overabundance of them, and by chewing them thoroughly you are making them much easier to digest. Because you'll be eating a reduced amount of food, you'll be losing weight, and because you are chewing your food thoroughly, you'll be saving energy in the digestion and elimination process, and you'll be storing that saved energy for your use.

How long can you keep this up? As mentioned, you can do this for several days, or you can do this pretty much forever as your regular diet. Eating wholesome and nutritious foods, eating moderate amounts of them, and chewing them well is the foundation of any good diet.

You can also try a reduced calorie diet for a time that provides some of the benefits of a fast but without as much stress on the body. My favorite is called the Metabolism Reset Diet, and it has recently been formulated and published by my favorite nutritional doctor and health writer, Alan Christianson. Dr. C., as he's fondly referred to by his clients and colleagues, has a wonderful gift of possessing a huge wealth of knowledge, understanding, and wisdom of all matters health and nutrition. And then he takes all that information, synthesizes it, and explains it in the most delightful and easy-to-understand way.

In January, 2019, Dr. C. released his book, *The Metabolism Reset Diet*. I'll provide a brief overview of this diet:

The Metabolism Reset Diet is not a permanent diet. It's designed to last 28 days, or less, and to be done once or periodically. As indicated by the name, the diet resets your metabolism. What does that mean and how does it work?

Your metabolism refers to how well your body processes energy. A person with a strong metabolism can delay or even skip meals and have enough strength to continue to work and play. A person with a weak metabolism not only can't delay or skip meals, but must eat between meals, and perhaps do so several times between each meal, just to keep going.

Why can one person skip meals and the other need to eat frequently to keep functioning? The answer is the health of the metabolism. Here's what is going on in the body of the healthy person: When that person eats, the body uses some fuel immediately, and it stores the excess energy as fuel (glycogen) in the liver and muscles for later use. When those stores are needed in the absence of food, the body easily retrieves them to use as energy. Again, that's what happens when the metabolism is strong, where the digestive system, liver, and muscles are all in tune and work in harmony to supply energy.

Here's what happens, or rather doesn't happen, in the person with a weak metabolism: The excess energy may or may not be stored in the liver, which may be damaged or clogged and "fatty." If the energy is not stored, there's nothing to retrieve when it's needed. But even if it is stored, a liver that is not working properly or in tune with the body will not release the stored energy as needed. In either case, the person will lack energy and will need to obtain energy from another source, which, much too often, is a sugary food that will only aggravate the problem.

And here's the beauty of the Metabolism Reset Diet: It provides just enough fuel to keep you going, but it has a strong effect on the liver, both cleaning and healing it for the duration of the reset. Once that occurs, the metabolism will be stronger and most of the energy issues will be resolved.

I highly recommend the Metabolism Reset Diet and, really, anything that Dr. Christianson teaches. In the world of health and nutrition, as far as I'm concerned, he is brilliant and he's genius number one.

22. Avoid Fad Diets

Pritikin, Atkins, South Beach, Raw Foods Only, Fruitarian, Mono, Rotation, Keto, High Protein, High Carb, Low Carb, and the like are all fad diets. And they are all virtually defunct. Okay, Keto is now wildly popular, but so were many of those other diets in their heyday. In time, people on those diets came to realize that while there may have seemed to be immediate benefits from those diets, long term, they were difficult to stay on and they were seriously flawed as to the principles of sound nutrition. Keto is on the same course. The Keto diet may seem to offer some immediate health benefits, but as many have found out, all fad diets, including Keto, are not healthy, sustainable diets. (See my book *The Keto Diet Damaged Our Health: A Better Approach*.)

What makes a diet a fad diet? It's one that seems to spring up out of nowhere, that is popular for a time, and then, usually within a few years to maybe a decade, fades and vanishes away. Fad diets all place an undue emphasis on one or more aspects of nutrition, and they all tend to villainize others.

Experts in the field of nutrition have given much advice as to what constitutes a healthy diet. Among those experts, there is one common thread, and this thread has endured decades of fad diets and other crazy eating notions. What is that thread? Our diets should be based on foods that are healthy, unprocessed, and in their natural state as much as possible. Eat a wide variety of nutritious foods for better health.

You may recall that I mentioned in the introduction of this book that I believe that humans and the Earth were created as a perfect match for each other. The variety of foods on this planet is almost mind-boggling. And those foods contain an abundance of colors, sizes, shapes, textures, aromas, and flavors, as well as an abundance of macronutrients (proteins, carbs, and fats), and an abundance of micronutrients (vitamins and minerals).

If such a large variety of foods and nutrients were supplied for our enjoyment and health needs, does it really make any sense to designate one or more of those food groups as villains and then severely restrict them from your diet?

Take, for example, dietary fat. Dietary fat has been viewed in ways that are all over the map—and most often very inaccurate. One view is that fats are bad, eat as little as possible. Another view is keto, stuff your face with as much fat as you can. One more view: Eating fat is what adds fat to your body. All of these views are incorrect. The balanced view is to enjoy fat in your diet, but don't eat too much of it. It's not only necessary, but it's a vital component to a healthy diet . . . but as with all other things, in moderation.

The Mediterranean diet that I mention in this book is not a fad diet. Why? Because it's based on sound nutritional principles. It includes healthful foods and a wide variety of them. It's balanced, it's reasonable, and it works. Therefore, the Mediterranean diet, or at least the principles of that diet, will endure for a very long time and should grow in popularity. Because it is the opposite of a fad diet, the Mediterranean diet and its principles of good nutrition will never fade away.

23. Consider a High-Speed Blender

A blender is an excellent, yet often overlooked, kitchen and dietary tool. The first blender was invented in 1922, but sales seemed to soar in the 1960s. No longer a luxury item, a blender could be found in almost any home.

You can buy a cheap blender for about $30, or a good blender for about $70. But if you are really into improving your health, and it won't strain your budget, I'd recommend splurging on an excellent, top-of-the-line, high-speed blender. We use ours every day, and it's provided a huge boost to our diet and health.

Some of these blenders retail for about $100, but the very best ones, the ones that commercial establishments use to make smoothies and other treats, sell for $400 or so.

Look for names such as Vitamix, Blendtec, Ninja, Nutribullet, and maybe one or two others.

Is there a king of blenders? I think so. The Vitamix is an amazingly versatile and powerful machine, and it's used by such major corporations as Whole Foods and nearly every other health food store I've ever been in. There are several models to choose from.

Some prefer Blendtec to Vitamix. In all fairness, I've never owned a Blendtec, but some who I trust would not be without one.

What can these top-of-the-line blenders do? First of all, they make remarkable smoothies. But they also make nut milks, such as almond and cashew. They make nut butters too. You can make soups right in your blender. When I say "make" soups, I don't mean mix the ingredients in the blender and then transfer the mix to the stove for cooking. You can actually cook the soup right in the blender. When run on high for a few minutes, the friction of those powerful blades creates a hot, creamy, delightful soup.

Using a high-speed blender, your opportunities to create are almost endless. You can add any variety of produce and fresh herbs and spices you like to create your drink. You can also add protein powders, spirulina, resistant starch, chia or flax seeds, and so much more.

Foods mixed in high-speed blenders retain their full amount of pulp, they are easy to digest (those blades "chew" way better than you ever could), and they keep in the refrigerator for up to two days.

Many people struggle to eat a sufficient amount of vegetables each day, and especially raw vegetables. Many find that they can easily consume their daily allotment when they do so in smoothies. (Parents, take note.)

One huge delight of the top-of-the-line blenders is the ease, and I really mean ease, of assembly and cleanup. Our Vitamix assembles in about two seconds, and the cleanup takes about a minute. To assemble, simply put the lid on. To clean, fill the Vitamix a little more than half way with warm or hot water, add 2-3 drops of dish soap, and then run on high for 30-60 seconds, rinse, and you are done. There's no need to disassemble and reassemble anything. Aside from the removable lid, the Vitamix stays as an intact unit.

What About Juicers?

Juicers have their place too. Some people have both a high-speed-blender and a juicer. If you were to buy only one, for most people, I'd suggest the blender, which is much more versatile and lets you enjoy the benefits of the healthful pulp. However, for those who like fresh juice, I can offer the following information: There are two main types of juicers: masticating and centrifugal. Masticating juicers are more expensive, but they yield higher quality juice. They extract the juice at a much lower rate of speed, and they are by far the best juicers for such items as grasses (wheat grass, etc.) and leafy greens. Centrifugal juicers are less expensive and they juice more produce in a shorter amount of time. For this reason, juice bars tend to use centrifugal juicers. Expect to pay about $150 for a good centrifugal juicer, and about $275 for a good masticating juicer. If there is a top name in masticating juicers, the nod likely goes to Omega.

But please, no matter what you decide about a juicer, if you can, invest in a good blender. It can make a huge difference in your kitchen and to your health and life.

The Best Way to Eat, Recap

Here's a recap of the main points of the preceding dietary chapters of this book: Eat a wide a variety of natural foods, including a colorful array of produce. Incorporate many living foods and fermented foods in your diet. Drink plenty of water. Avoid foods that are unhealthful, such as refined carbohydrates and fried and excess saturated fats. Avoid foods with chemicals, overly processed foods, and foods you may be allergic to.

Eat a high protein, low-carbohydrate breakfast, eat healthful snacks as needed, and consider cycling your carbohydrates, which means eating smaller amounts in the morning for breakfast and more at lunch and even more at dinner.

Chew your foods thoroughly, which brings many health benefits, especially to your blood sugar levels, your digestion, and your gut health. Don't overeat, and keep plenty of healthful foods on hand.

To the extent you do these things, to that extent your health will improve. The idea is to give your body all it needs and to avoid what will harm or burden it. By doing this, all systems of your body will be in position to flourish, including your heart, muscles, liver, brain, and all of your organs.

Eating correctly makes a huge difference!

The World's Healthiest Diet

24. The Mediterranean Diet

The best diet in the world would be one that is tailored especially for you, to meet your exact nutritional requirements. Such a diet is, of course, mostly unrealistic. But by starting with a healthy foundation, and making adjustments from there, you can come close. Which diet is the healthiest foundation for the majority of health seekers?

The *U.S. News and World Report* assembled a team of experts to study and rank the top 40 best-known diets. In the categories of Best Diet for Healthy Eating and Best Diet Overall, which was crowned the healthiest? The Mediterranean diet. This diet is based on the lifestyles of the healthiest people of the Mediterranean region, which includes parts of such countries as Italy, France, Spain, Greece, Morocco, and Portugal. The key feature of the diet is to eat natural, unprocessed foods as your dietary staple. Such foods as vegetables, fruits, olive oil, beans, nuts, seeds, grains, herbs, and spices form the bulk of the diet. Fish and seafood should be eaten often, at least two times a week. Moderate portions of poultry, eggs, cheese, and yogurt can be eaten daily or weekly. Meats, such as beef and pork, and sweets should be eaten sparingly, if at all.

Additionally, the Mediterranean diet stresses such non-dietary issues as spending time with friends, eating meals together, relaxing together, and engaging in healthful physical activity.

It's clear from the above description that the Mediterranean diet is natural and healthy. There is an abundance of good books on the market that explain the diet in detail.

48   Better Health: Happier Living

You may find the Mediterranean Diet Pyramid, below, helpful. You can order a poster of the pyramid, download a free PDF, or even order a magnet to stick on your refrigerator. Thus, every time you open that door you'll be reminded of the importance of eating in this healthful and enjoyable way. For posters, PDFs, and magnets, contact Oldways, a non-profit organization that is dedicated to teaching people how to eat a healthier, more natural diet, at www.oldwayspt.org/medpyramid.

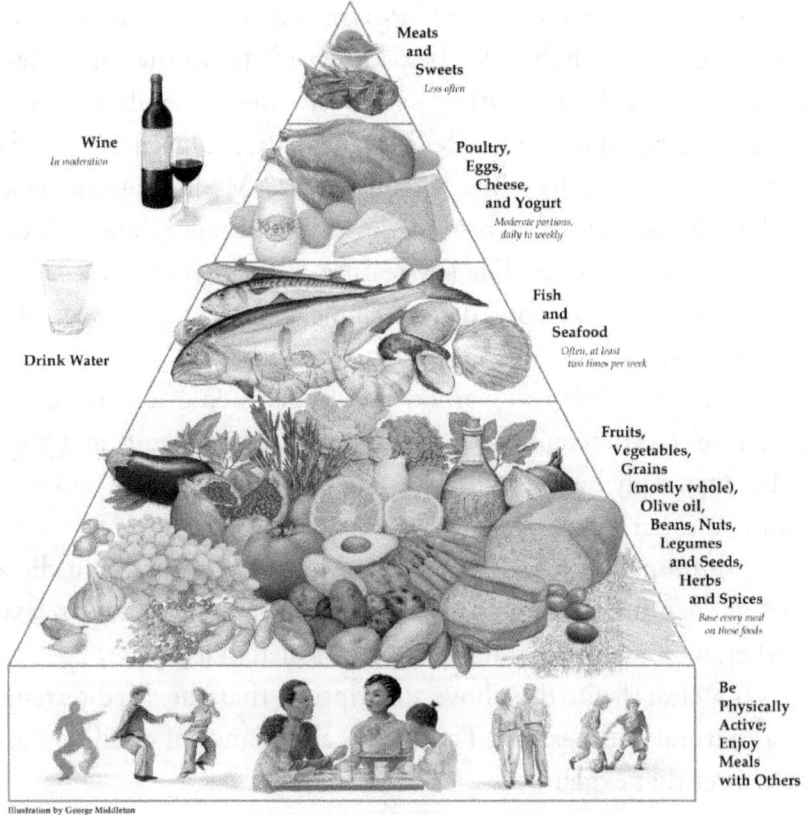

25. Guidelines to Enhance the Mediterranean Diet

As wonderful as the Mediterranean diet is, and as helpful as the Mediterranean diet food pyramid is, most people would benefit from guidance regarding how to use the pyramid and how to make the diet their own. For instance, while eating according to the pyramid, it is very possible that one could be eating too many fruits and grains (which are at the base of the pyramid) and not enough vegetables (which are also at the base of the pyramid). The pyramid doesn't make a distinction, but your body does.

The guidelines in this section will ensure that you are eating the most balanced and healthful diet possible. Many of the principles have been explained in previous chapters of this book, but I'll give a recap here as well as provide additional information that will help you tailor your diet to your specific needs and preferences.

We'll start at the base of the pyramid and work are way up:

The Bottom Layer (Activities): The bottom layer—the non-dietary layer—of the pyramid is just about perfect. It's best to engage in these activities every day if possible, according to your circumstances. The second half of this book, under the section Additional Paths to Better Health, corresponds to this layer. You can find many ways to excel at this layer in those chapters.

The Fruits, Vegetables, Grains, Olive Oil, Beans, Nuts, Legumes, Seeds, Herbs, and Spices Layer: This layer is loaded with the foods that should make up the majority of your diet. Please note these helpful guidelines:

Limit **fruits** to perhaps 2-3 servings daily. Fruits are excellent, nutrient-rich, cleansing foods. But they also tend to be high in sugar content. It's best to eat only small-to-moderate amounts of fruit at one time. By eating fruits along with foods that contain proteins and fats, you'll slow the absorption of sugar, which leads to a steadier flow of energy.

You can exceed the 2-3 limit of fruits if you primarily eat fruits that do not have a high sugar content, such as grapefruit, lemons, limes, berries, avocados (yes, it's a fruit), and the like. You can also eat additional fruit if you are very active physically: manual laborers and athletes fall into this category.

Eat a minimum of 4-6 servings of **vegetables** daily. Vegetables are also nutrient-rich foods, and they tend to be lower in sugar than fruits. It's best to eat at least a couple of those servings raw. Green leafy vegetables, such as lettuce, are normally eaten raw, and they are packed with important, health-building nutrients.

Starchy vegetables, such as potatoes, sweet potatoes, and yams, are all healthful foods. But due to their high carbohydrate content, it's best to eat them in moderation. One or two daily servings should be enough for most people.

Grains are a little trickier, as allergies to various grains, especially wheat and corn, are prevalent. So be sure to eat grains that you are not allergic or sensitive to. Consider adding fat content, such as olive oil, some seeds, or a little butter, to your grains. The fats will slow down the absorption of the carbohydrates, which will regulate your blood sugar levels and prevent glucose and insulin spikes. If you believe you are allergic or sensitive to gluten, be sure to eat gluten-free grains. And as the pyramid indicates, make sure to eat whole grains.

Olive oil, which is a major dietary staple of the Mediterranean region, is both a luxurious treat and a superfood at the same time. Of course, olive oil is very high in fat (though healthful fat), and should therefore be eaten in moderation. A couple of tablespoons a day on average could be about right for most people. And make sure to buy extra virgin olive oil (EVOO), which is produced by pressing the olives and extracting their juice. Other grades of olive oils are extracted through a chemical process, and you want to keep your chemical intake as low as possible.

There's some controversy about the healthfulness of **beans**. To this, I say poppycock. Beans are a wonderful source of protein, healthful carbohydrates, fiber, vitamins, and minerals. Beans, and especially their liquid, called aquafaba (which means, literally, "water of beans"), are high in resistant starch, which brings health benefits of its own. Of course, I'm referring to beans such as white beans (navy, great northern, cannellini), pinto beans, black beans, and so on. Baked beans, ranch beans, and other such prepared beans, those with added sugars, should be avoided. If you feel you must eat them, even for an occasional splurge, it's best to drain as much of the sugary liquid as possible.

Nuts and seeds are both powerhouses of nutritional energy. Sadly though, most people neglect to make these little marvels a part of their daily diets.

There are many nut and seed varieties to choose from, but perhaps the most widely available nuts are almonds, cashews, walnuts, pecans, macadamias, pistachio, Brazil nuts, and pine nuts; and the most widely available seeds are sunflower, sesame, chia ("ch-ch-ch-chia"), flax, and pumpkin. Peanuts are not on the list of nuts or seeds because technically they are a legume. And, by the way, quinoa (pronounced *keen-wa*) should be on the list, because quinoa is a seed, but it has the characteristics of a grain and is most often viewed as a grain by the public. Quinoa, which has become very popular in recent years, is an excellent source of nutrition.

Make sure that the nuts and seeds you buy are fresh, not rancid. Rancid nuts and seeds can usually be detected by smell or taste. They will not only taste bad, but eating them can lead to health issues.

Bulk seeds and nuts are the most likely to be rancid. It's impossible to tell how long they've been sitting in that bin. Packaged nuts and seeds are likely to be fresh if they are unopened and the expiration date has not arrived. However, once they've been opened and exposed to air, they can become rancid before the expiration date.

Nuts and seeds are best consumed, if possible, raw and unsalted.

Legumes are a little harder to classify, and if you research the topic, you'll probably find some conflicting and confusing information. For instance, some consider green beans and peas to be legumes, while others consider them vegetables. For simplicity sake, let's just say that common legumes include such crops as peas, garbanzo beans (chickpeas), peanuts, soybeans, lentils, carob, and alfalfa. It's pretty easy to see where some of the confusion comes in, because while nuts and beans are not legumes, some legumes include the words "nuts" and "beans" in their names: pea**nuts**, garbanzo **beans**, soy**beans**. (The English language . . . it doesn't always make cents scents sense.)

And as strange and confusing as the categorization of legumes is, pronouncing the word is probably just as strange and confusing, as well as awkward and perhaps irritating. There are two correct ways to pronounce legume: leg-yoom and le'gyoom, Many incorrectly pronounce it le'goom.

Legumes, no matter how you classify them, or how you pronounce them, are excellent dietary staples.

The Fish and Seafood Layer: Seafood is an excellent source of protein, and I agree that it should be eaten at least a couple of times a week if possible. Make sure the seafood is fresh—the smell-test is much better than asking the clerk, who seems almost programmed to say "it just came in this morning" no matter what that fish looks and smells like. And even if the fish did "come in" that morning, there's a more important question that the clerk will not know the answer to: When was it caught? Again, the smell-test is your best defense.

Wild caught fish is superior to "farmed" fish, and fresh fish is better than frozen fish. What about canned fish? Actually, not so bad. Canned tuna, salmon, kippers, and the like can be handy sources of protein and they can get you out of some tight jams, such as when the refrigerator is running near empty or your schedule is over packed. If possible, though, make fresh fish your staple for this layer.

The Poultry, Eggs, Cheese, and Yogurt Layer: This might be called the "controversy layer," as the foods in this layer are probably more controversial than in the other layers.

Poultry is generally accepted by most dietary experts as being healthy, but eggs and dairy products are subject to a wide range of opinions. Therefore, it's probably a good thing that this layer is not at the base of the pyramid.

Poultry, and in particular chicken, is an excellent staple in many diets. Sadly, chickens are usually kept in deplorable conditions: they are overcrowded in cages, have no room to roam, and are stuffed with hormones and antibiotics. This makes for a stressed and sick animal, and a sick animal is never a good dietary choice.

Thankfully, there are viable options. Free-range chicken is now more readily available. Free-range chickens are not caged; they are able to roam. Obviously, this makes for a healthier chicken. Better yet are free-range chickens that have never been fed antibiotics. These are often referred to as "organic" chickens, and they are a superior choice. Major companies like Perdue are now selling both free-range and organic chicken.

Eggs are also the subject of much controversy. On the one hand, they have been touted as the perfect food. On the other, they are villainized as cholesterol-raising troublemakers. In reality, they are probably somewhere between those two extremes.

Eggs are subject to many of the same concerns I mentioned about eating chicken meat. Chickens that are stressed and sickly and glutted with antibiotics are probably not laying the highest-quality eggs. You can see evidence of that in the color of the yolks, which are often a pale shade of yellow.

Several companies are now selling eggs that are harvested from free-range chickens or organic chickens. These eggs are quite a bit more costly than the lower-quality eggs. Is the extra cost worth it? For many, yes. You can see the difference in the yolks, which are usually a brighter, richer, healthier looking color, sometimes even bordering on orange. Depending upon your budget and preferences, you may want to consider free-range or organic eggs. Look for names like Eggland's Best and others.

You may have noticed that eggs have either white or brown shells. Nutritionally, does it matter which you buy? No. One is not a healthier choice than the other. The color of the shell depends on the type of chicken that produced the egg. Some chicken breeds lay white eggs (Andulusian, Leghorn), others lay brown eggs (Sussex, Rhode Island Red). There's probably not a noticeable difference in taste. It's just a matter of personal preference. Note: Some chicken breeds lay other color eggs, such as green, blue, cream colored, etc.

Interesting Note: Many years ago, almost all eggs that were marketed had white shells. In perhaps the 1970s, brown eggs began to be marketed and they gained immediate popularity. Why? It seems that they benefited from the early stages of the health food era, where anything brown was considered superior. Brown sugar was considered healthier than white sugar, brown rice than white rice, whole wheat (brown) flour over white flour, so naturally (or maybe oddly) many assumed that brown eggs are superior nutritionally to white eggs.

Dairy products are also very controversial. Some make the argument that no other animal continues to eat dairy products after they are weaned. Others make the argument that dairy products are good sources of nutrition and an excellent way to add taste and variety to our diets. Which side is correct? They both are. I can't argue with either one of those statements.

So here's what I believe is a balanced way of looking at the matter . . . If you want to eat dairy products and if you are not allergic to them or the lactose in them, go ahead and enjoy them. As the pyramid indicates, eat no more than moderate portions of dairy daily to weekly. (Remember, we are pretty close to the top of the pyramid now, so dairy should not be a main staple.) Be sure to eat only high-quality dairy products. For instance, if buying yogurt, skip the ultra-sweet stuff and brands made with artificial ingredients. Grass-fed milk, if available, is a superior choice.

The Top Layer (Meats and Sweets): Indeed, eat these foods sparingly, if at all.

I don't consider meats and sweets to be in the same category. You can make a case that high-quality grass-fed beef is a health food.

Foods high in sugar and high-fructose corn syrup? No case there at all. So I give the nod to meats over sweets.

Commercial **beef** is not what it used to be. Scientists have learned how to get that cattle beefy and fat and to do it quick. Thus, instead of letting the cattle roam contentedly in fields and feed on grass, they are kept in stalls and fed grains, growth hormones, and antibiotics. Many believe that such meat is not fit for human consumption.

Is there a reasonable alternative? Yes, there is. And as usual, it involves going back to square one. In this case, that means letting cattle roam contentedly in fields and feed on the grass. What a novel idea! So look for beef that is labeled "grass-fed" or "grass-finished." It's a bit more expensive, but it's definitely a more natural meat and healthier.

Pork's nutritional reputation has been all over the map, but mostly it's been villainized. Some have viewed pork as a trichinosis-ridden slab on a plate. The pork industry, on the other hand, has labeled and marketed pork as "the other white meat." By doing so, it has tried to assign pork the same prized status as chicken in the public's mind. As with so many controversies, the truth is somewhere in the middle between the two extremes. Pork is really not that bad, but it's also not that good. Pork, if eaten at all, is best eaten in moderate amounts and not as a main staple in the diet. And please, make sure pork is cooked to the recommended temperature.

If you decide to eat **sweets**, do so wisely. Strive to eat the healthiest sweet that will satisfy you. For instance, a sweet potato or yam with a little brown sugar is a better desert choice than a double-decker chocolate-lava-bomb-volcano. Of course, if you decide to have the sweet potato or yam with honey instead of sugar, or just by itself, that's even better.

Can you be a vegetarian or a vegan on the Mediterranean diet? Yes, you can, if that is your desire. Vegetarians, and especially vegans, will be eating foods mostly from the base layer of the diet.

Therefore, it's important that they make sure to eat enough of the higher protein foods in that layer, such as beans, legumes, nuts, and seeds. A high-quality, vegetable-based protein powder may be useful in meeting daily protein needs.

A few more dietary suggestions:

- It is important to cook all meats to the proper temperature. Cooking with a meat thermometer not only drastically reduces any risk of food-borne illness, but it's also an effective way to ensure that your meat is cooked according to your taste preference.

- Meat should not comprise the main part of the meal. A huge steak with a tiny portion of asparagus is not a good dinner. Vegetables should normally dominate your plate. Try to keep meat portions small, normally four to six ounces or less.

- Water is listed at the side of the pyramid, because technically water is not a food. (Zero calories.) But as mentioned earlier in this book, it's important to drink sufficient amounts of water daily.

Additional Paths to Better Health

Our health is clearly linked to our dietary patterns. But our health is also deeply affected by so many other matters: How we exercise our bodies and minds, how we sleep, how we deal with stress, how we think, how we view and treat others, how we view ourselves, how we laugh, and many others.

This section will help you to seriously boost your health status and well-being by teaching you tried-and-true methods of good, sound, logical living.

26. Exercise Your Body

"Each time you exercise, you come back stronger. Before long, you get flat-out tough. Both mentally and physically." – Rafer Johnson, Olympic Gold Medalist

It's very evident that our bodies were designed to move, to move in a variety of ways, and to do so often. You have the capacity to walk, to run, to jump, to swim, to lift, to skip, to bend, to hop, to stretch. (At least, you likely had those as a youth, but you might have lost some capacity along the way.) When you follow a routine involving some or most of those activities, your body stays tuned and toned. Or as Rafer Johnson, who was once considered the "world's best athlete," said, "you get flat-out tough."

There are three main categories of exercise. They are cardio, resistance, and stretching. There's also play. I'll give a brief overview of each of these.

Stretching. Our muscles, tendons, and ligaments all need to be stretched on a regular basis. If they are not, they tend to shorten and stiffen. That makes them more susceptible to injury. For that reason, and because stretching is calming and feels good, stretching is highly beneficial.

Here's a few tips to enhance your stretching and to make it most advantageous:

1. Start slowly: Don't begin an exercise session with a hard stretch. Your muscles are not ready for that yet. Ease your way into your session. And consider warming up with a walk before you begin to stretch.

2. Don't bounce. Bouncing has been found to elicit a defensive reaction in the muscles that makes them tighten rather than loosen. Especially is bouncing undesirable when the muscles are "cold" and have not been warmed by walking or light running.

3. Don't overstretch. Muscles that are overstretched can stiffen, pull, and tear. This does not feel very good! Proper stretches, however, do feel good and are very relaxing.

4. Do stretch gently. Stretch to a comfortable position, hold that position for about 20-30 seconds, and then release. If during the stretch you feel strain or pain and a need to back off a little, do so. On the other hand, if going a little further feels safe, feel free to go ahead. Keep paying attention to how each stretch feels, and adjust accordingly.

5. Do not start your new stretching session at the same level you left off your previous one; you must begin gently and work into each session anew. I fall into this trap from time to time: If during a stretching session I am able to comfortably touch my wrist to my toes, the next time I stretch, even a day or more later, I almost automatically want to start at that same level. My mind is game for it, my body is not; and that entire stretching session is not really pleasant or beneficial. Rather, always stretch to the proper limit on every stretch in every session; by doing this you will benefit the most from your session and will reduce any chance of pain or injury. Likely, after you've stretched gently for a few minutes, you'll begin to limber up and be able to safely stretch further.

6. Finally, here's a tip from my chiropractor: Consider stretching one leg at a time. I learned this the hard way, as my deep stretching sessions were resulting in lower back misalignment and pain. (Which was the exact opposite result of what I was striving for.) Dr. V. said that when I sit on the floor and touch my toes, I should do one leg at a time. When you grab both feet and get into a good stretch, you are putting tremendous torque on your lower spine. In my case, I was literally pulling it out of joint. I took his advice and have not had the problem since.

Cardio. Cardio, of course, refers to the heart. In moderation, the heart, along with the lungs, thrive from a good aerobic workout.

We all know what flabby muscles look like. The heart is a muscle, your most important muscle, and it too becomes "flabby" if it is not regularly exercised.

There are various types of cardio workouts. Anything with sustained motion that gets the heart beating faster for a moderate or extended period of time is cardio. Examples of cardio are walking, jogging, running, swimming, rowing, treadmill walking, stair climbing, sports with constant movement like soccer, and the like.

How hard should you exercise when doing cardio? One way to calculate this is by a combination of age and pulse rate. There are charts and formulas for this. But the simplest and perhaps most effective method is the "talk test." If you can no longer comfortably carry on a conversation while exercising, you've likely exceeded your cardio exercise limit. Every person is different, and every person has different needs and a different capacity, but for most, the best zone to be in is to exercise at a pace at or below the limit of where you can still comfortably carry on a conversation. If you have to huff and puff and gasp during the conversation, it's probably best to slow it down.

How long should you exercise when doing cardio? That's up to you: and it depends to a large degree on your level of fitness, the reason you exercise, and the amount of time you have to spend exercising. It's usually best to do at least 10 minutes of cardio. Some find 20-45 minutes an agreeable amount. And some like a long, slow walk every once in a while, perhaps on weekends, of an hour or more.

Some suggestions: Try not to walk on a busy road: noise, danger from vehicles, air pollution, and idiots can make your walk stressful and uncomfortable. Many feel safer bringing a dog-repellant spray. Have your cell phone handy (and charged, please). Walking with a friend can be helpful too.

What should you think about when you walk? You can work out your problems if you like, but if possible, pay attention to the fresh air and the beauty surrounding you.

Listening to music can be helpful. Scientific studies have proven that music helps us exercise longer and harder. We start moving to the music, and the exercise almost becomes secondary. Sometimes you'll extend your session just to hear that next song or two that you like so much.

Please notice this wonderful passage about music and exercise from an article published in *Scientific American* on March 20, 2013, written by Ferris Jabr.

"Research on the interplay of music and exercise dates to at least 1911, when American investigator Leonard Ayres found that cyclists pedaled faster while a band was playing than when it was silent. Since then psychologists have conducted around a hundred studies on the way music changes people's performance in a variety of physical activities, ranging in intensity from strolling to sprinting.

"In the last 10 years the body of research on workout music has swelled considerably, helping psychologists refine their ideas about why exercise and music are such an effective pairing for so many people as well as how music changes the body and mind during physical exertion. Music distracts people from pain and fatigue, elevates mood, increases endurance, reduces perceived effort and may even promote metabolic efficiency. When listening to music, people run farther, bike longer and swim faster than usual—often without realizing it. In a 2012 review of the research, Costas Karageorghis of Brunel University in London, one of the world's leading experts on the psychology of exercise music, wrote that one could think of music as 'a type of legal performance-enhancing drug.'"

Music or sans music, cardio is an excellent way to build heart and lung capacity.

Resistance. Resistance refers to pushing or pulling against objects with the goal of building muscle size, strength, tone, and endurance.

When I was a child, there were two main types of resistance exercises: isotonics and isometrics. Thankfully, we've come a long way. Isotonics essentially refer to weight lifting. Isometrics refer to pitting one muscle against the other or pushing or pulling against an immovable object. As an example, you'd clasp your hands and with one hand pull toward your body and the other hand push away. The theory was that you'd be exercising the biceps of one arm and the triceps of the other. In reality, it felt as though you were having a fight with yourself, and it hurt. It was an unnatural movement, a strain, and it gave me a headache. Today there are not only free weights, but resistance machines galore. Many of those machines are superb.

When using weights or resistance machines, keep these things in mind:

1. Unless you are a trained athlete or experienced weight lifter, don't push it to the limit. Don't try to lift more weight than you can comfortably handle. Begin slowly, and let your body adapt to your new routine.

2. Perform repetitions, in sets. Repetitions refer to how many times you've performed a movement during a particular lift. Each time that you begin an exercise, do a certain number of repetitions, and then stop, that's a set. For instance, if you pick up a barbell, curl it 10 times, and then you put it down, you've done one set of 10 repetitions of curls. Do that again, and you've done two sets of 10 repetitions.

3. Each set should push your muscles close to your limit, but not over your limit, to where you are seriously straining to finish. (Competitive athletes are a sometimes exception to this rule.) Therefore, your last two or three repetitions in a set should be difficult, but they should not require your all-out effort. When you feel like you could do one or two or maybe three more repetitions, but with tremendous strain, right there is where you should end the set. The expression "train, don't strain," is especially appropriate for resistance exercise.

4. You can decide how many sets to do of a certain exercise. Competitive lifters or body builders perform many sets, perhaps six or more, to shock their muscles to make them super big and strong. For most people, two or three sets of a lift should be about right. You can perform the sets in any order that you want to, but most find it

advantageous to do one exercise at a time, such as arm curls, and when they have completed all sets of those curls, they move on to the next exercise, such as leg extensions.

5. Consider starting with a lighter weight and increasing the amount of weight in subsequent sets. This allows the muscles to warm up at a lighter weight and get used to the movement before tackling a heavier weight. Here's a three-set example of how that could work: Bench Press: 1st set, 50 pounds x 12 repetitions; 2nd set, 60 pounds x 8 repetitions; 3rd set, 70 pounds x 5 repetitions.

Note: Here's another benefit from starting with a lighter weight and increasing to a heavier weight . . . Sometimes we may have a minor injury that we are not aware of or that we forgot about. Perhaps we have a slightly strained wrist that we pay no attention to. It's easy to ignore that wrist when going about the routine matters of life. But when you lift a heavy weight, you may be reminded of that injury in no uncertain terms with a quick shot of pain. It's safer to experience that pain with a lighter weight than a heavier one, and it's a signal to back off until the injury is healed.

6. Never train the same muscles on consecutive days. When you lift weights, your muscles are going through a two-step process. First, lifting actually breaks them down and "damages" them. Second, during the resting period that follows, the muscles rebuild and become stronger than they were before the workout.

That process takes about 48 hours. If you exercise the same muscle a day later, or 24 hours later, it has not had time to recover, strengthen, and rebuild from the previous workout. By doing so, you'd be risking injury and shortchanging your efforts to get stronger.

There are two ways you can ensure that you are not exercising the same muscles with weights two days in a row. 1. Don't lift weights on consecutive days. That's the most logical method for most of us. So if you want to work out, say, five days a week, you may lift weights on Monday, Wednesday, and Friday, and you may walk, play a sport, use the treadmill, and so forth, on Tuesday and Thursday. 2. Especially serious athletes and weightlifters may want to train with weights on consecutive days. Here's how they can make a success of that: They can alternate lifting days one of two ways. 1. They can do only upper body exercises one day and then lower body exercises the next day. 2. Or, they can do pushing exercises one day (bench press, military press, leg extension, leg press, etc.) and pulling exercises the next (arm curls, wrist curls, leg curls, rows, etc.) Either way, the same muscles are not being used to lift on consecutive days.

7. You may be wondering if you are better off lifting heavier weights with less repetitions or lighter weights with more repetitions. That depends on your goals and your preferences, and to some degree your age and physical condition. Heavier weights build bulk and strength. Lighter weights tone the muscles and give them more endurance. If there is a gender divide, men often prefer heavier weights with less repetitions, and woman often prefer lighter weights with more repetitions.

The middle point is somewhere around 10-12 repetitions per set. That's considered a good compromise between bulk and strength, and tone and endurance. Power athletes who need immediate bursts of strength, such as football players, may go as low as 2-5 repetitions per set. Those not interested in power or bulk but in a well-toned appearance may do 15-25 repetitions per set.

If you are performing multiple sets, a good compromise might be to start with a set of more than 10-12 reps, and then increase the weight and do less than 10-12 reps by the last set. This gives your muscles the best of both worlds. A three-set example of this follows: Bench Press, 1st set, 65 pounds, 16 reps; 2nd set, 80 pounds, 10 reps; 3rd set, 95 pounds, 6 reps.

8. Finally, remember to train, not strain. You want your exercise program to enhance your health, not injure you and undermine your health.

Note for Senior Citizens. As you grow older, your muscles lose size, strength, and endurance. A simple and moderate resistance training program, along with walking, is an excellent way to turn back the hands of time and enjoy youthful vigor well into your golden years. As my dear friend Emilee DeCelles has been known to say: "Growing old is not for sissies." Emilee not only talks the talk, but she walks the walk. She's one octogenarian who I would not want mad at me.

Play. And finally, there is good old play. While play doesn't fit neatly into any one category (cardio, strength, stretching), you can meet some of your exercise requirements by participating in many sports and games. For instance, if you enjoy sports like basketball or tennis, you'll likely be getting a good cardio workout.

Supplement your play with the other types of exercise. If you play basketball, you may or may not need additional cardio, but you will definitely benefit from strength training and stretching.

Finally, remember to have fun when you play; select a sport that you truly enjoy. After all, it's called "play" for a reason.

In summary, famed 20th-century football coach Bud Wilkinson once described football as "22 on the field, badly in need of rest, and 40,000 in the stands, badly in need of exercise." He made a good point. We badly need some exercise to feel our best and to live our best. If you make sure to get sufficient exercise, you will enhance your life in many ways, including physically, mentally, emotionally, and perhaps socially.

Medical Note: Exercise is universally acknowledged as a health-building activity. However, it's recommended that you consult with your physician before beginning any new exercise program. Each person has a different body makeup as well as different medical needs and limitations.

27. Exercise Your Brain (Stay Mentally Sharp)

The human brain has been described as the most complex object in the entire universe. And rightly so, because the depth of its complexity is astonishing; there are literally millions of finely-tuned processes taking place every second in your brain.

And while the brain is not a muscle (it's an organ), it has something in common with every muscle in your body . . . to function properly, it needs lots of exercise.

How can you exercise your brain? Simply put, use it. You are using it right now by reading. Reading is great for the brain. Other ways to exercise your brain are by engaging in tasks that put your mind to the test: playing puzzles like Sudoku, learning a new language, learning about a new subject, learning to use a computer, learning to program a computer, thinking deeply about things, and so on.

Do you need to max out your brain to properly exercise it? Of course not; you don't have to study nuclear physics. Suggesting that would be like telling someone they needed to run 25 miles every day to properly exercise their body. They don't.

Exercising your brain, just as exercising your body, should be fun. You can play entertaining games such as checkers or chess, or you can even read material that is light in nature. Even reading humorous material, or reading witty cartoons, can stretch, strengthen, and tune your brain. Notice how these two cartoons get your brain working in a subtle and pleasant way.

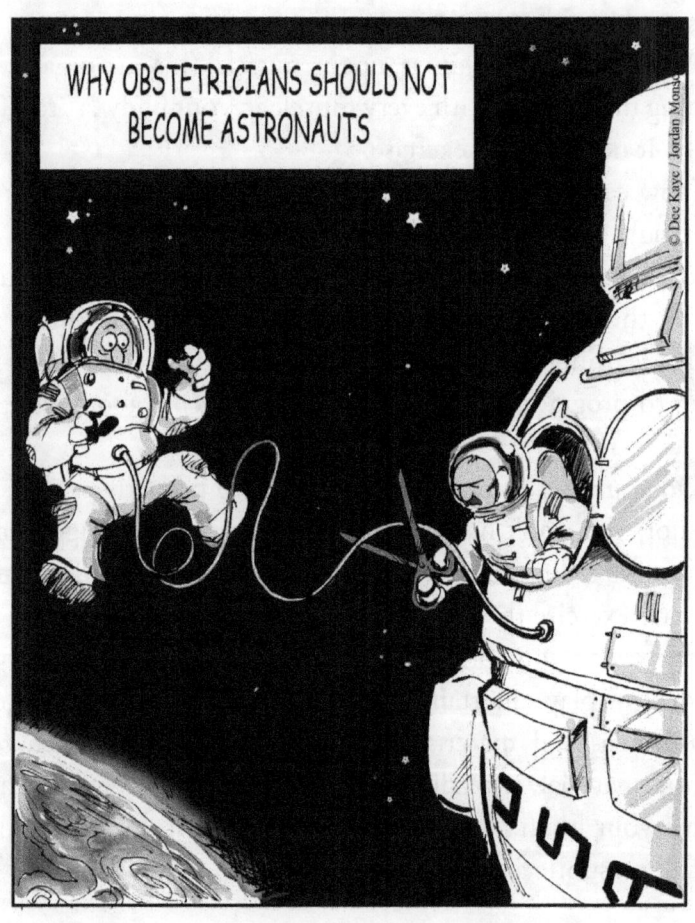

Additional Paths to Better Health 69

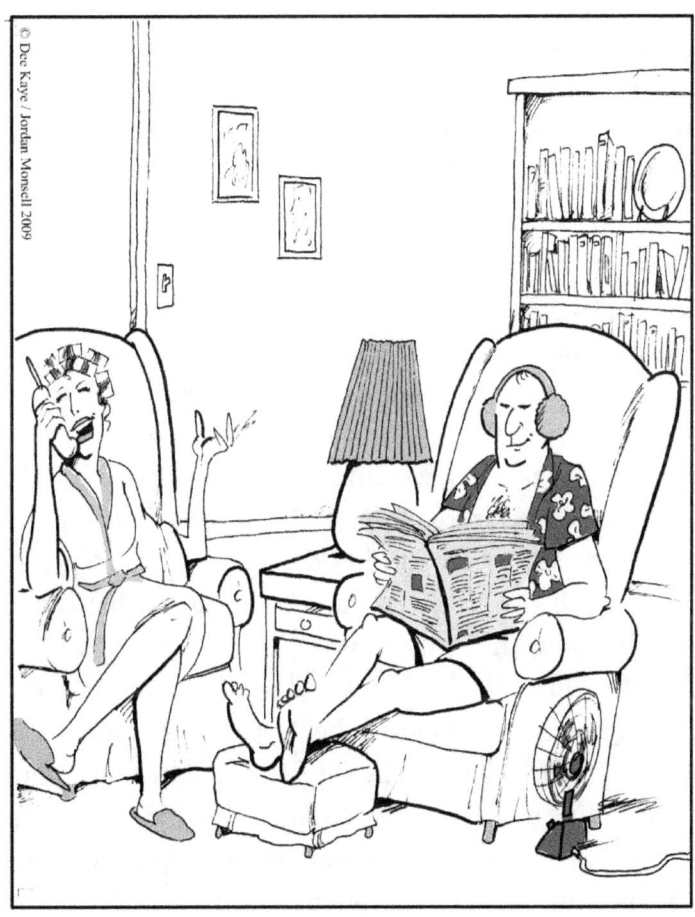

"Oh, and Roger developed a strange condition where he feels cold on evenings and weekends, oh, and . . ."

Sometimes brain-teasing questions can build a more powerful brain. Try to come up with the answer to this rather simple but somehow complex equation: A man was working in his office, when another man stopped by to visit him. After a time, the visitor left, and a colleague asked the worker who it was that came to see him. The worker responded by saying: "A brother and sister I have none; but that man's father is my father's son." Can you decipher the answer?

Or, try this one: A man and his son are driving and they are involved in a terrible accident. The father dies immediately, and the boy is taken to a medical center by ambulance. He is hurt badly, and he requires surgery. The surgeon takes a look at the boy and says: "I can't operate on this boy. He's my son." Who is the surgeon?

Learning new facts is very enjoyable and also a brain-building activity. For instance, did you know that polar bears are excellent swimmers, and they can swim for up to 200 miles at one time? Or did you know that as water gets colder, it gets more dense and heavier? But once the temperature drops to 39 degrees (Fahrenheit), the opposite occurs, and water gets less dense and lighter until it freezes at 32 degrees. This is no trivial matter, as this is what causes ice to form on the top of the body of water and what prevents bodies of water from freezing completely solid, thus destroying all life in them. Or do you know how to locate the North Star, which is a star of ordinary size and brightness? The Big Dipper, which is easy to locate, always points directly to the North Star, and it does so even when the Dipper, which rotates in the sky, is sideways or upside down. Finally, do you know why the moon is often lit in two different ways? The illuminated part is bright, but the other part is only slightly illuminated? The bright part is the sun's light directly hitting the moon, but the slightly lit part is illuminated by the light of the sun that has hit the Earth and then reflected to the moon. This is called "Earthshine."

And while we're discussing the moon, here is one more fascinating fact: The sun is 400 times further away from the Earth than the moon. Now, here is a question: How many times bigger than

Additional Paths to Better Health 71

the moon is the sun? The answer becomes obvious once every blue moon—that's just a saying—but in reality, the answer becomes obvious every full solar eclipse. Now that I've mentioned that, try to figure out how many times bigger the sun is than the moon. The answer is provided at the end of this chapter.

It's also fun to learn about oddities in the world around us. For instance, did you know that a clock in Pensacola, Florida, correctly reads the same exact time as it does in Vale, Oregon? But you may think, wait a moment, that's not possible. Florida is on the Atlantic Coast and Oregon is on the Pacific Coast. That's correct, but Pensacola, in the Florida Panhandle, is in the Central Time zone, and Vale, near the Idaho border, is in the Mountain Time zone. So for one hour each year, when the clock has "fallen back" an hour in Pensacola and not yet done so in Vale, the local time in those two cities is exactly the same.

Even optical illusions can be a mental challenge. For instance, what do you see in the image below?

Do you see a series of black horizontal bars and a series of white horizontal bars? And are those bars interrupted by three smaller light gray bars on the left side and also three darker gray bars on the right side.

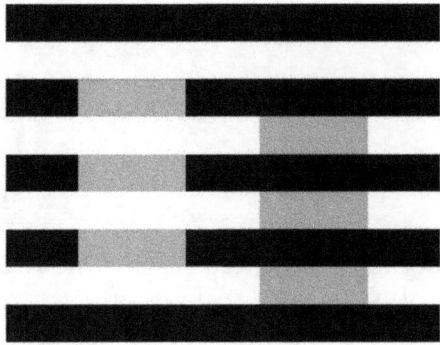

If you are seeing this, you are seeing it incorrectly. (Don't worry about that; everyone sees it incorrectly.) So what is really there? It may surprise you to learn that the light gray bars to the left and the dark gray bars to the right are really not what they seem. Rather, they are both the same exact shade of gray. I know, you just looked at the graphic again and find that hard to believe, because your eyes are telling you something different. But here's what's happening . . . the gray bars to the left look lighter than they are because they are on a dark (black) background; and the three gray bars to the right look lighter than they are because they are on a light (white) background.

Another way to exercise your brain—and in the process combine bodily exercise—is by playing sports that require strategy. Tennis, for example, is filled with constant decisions as to where to hit the ball, how hard to hit it, where to position yourself on the court, whether or not to approach the net, what type of spin to put on the ball, and so forth. Even keeping score can provide somewhat of a mental workout.

Especially do older people need to exercise their brains. Time will shrink and slow the connections, and mental exercise is a great way to combat that.

Question: What do the two images below have in common?

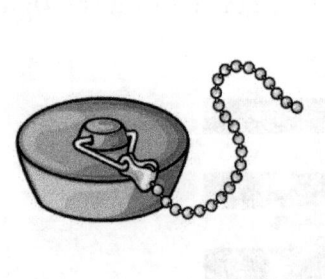
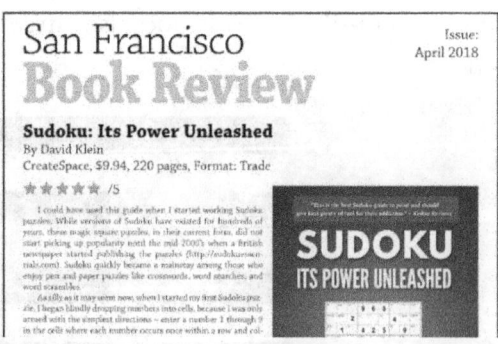

Answer: They are both cheap plugs. One is a cheap plug for a bathroom sink, and the other is a cheap plug for my award-winning Sudoku book, *Sudoku: Its Power Unleashed*. Mental activity like Sudoku keeps the brain active and supple.

Your brain is a marvel. Appreciate it, use it, and build it. It will serve you very well if you do.

Answer to the visitor question: The man's son was the visitor. ("My father's son" is me or one of my brothers. But I don't have a brother or sister, so it has to be me. Reworded then, "That man's father is me.")

Answer to the surgeon question: The surgeon is his mother.

Answer to the sun-moon quiz: The sun is 400 times larger than the moon. Because it is 400 times larger, and also 400 times further away, that is why the moon fits perfectly over the sun during a full solar eclipse.

28. Maintain Your Proper Body Weight (And Shape)

Notice this extraordinary opening to a June 12, 2015 report in the *Washington Post*, by staff writer Christopher Ingraham:

"The average American woman weighs 166.2 pounds, according to the Centers for Disease Control and Prevention. As *reddit* recently pointed out, that's almost exactly as much as the average American man weighed in the early 1960s. Men, you're not looking too hot in this scenario either. Over the same time period you gained nearly 30 pounds, from 166.3 in the 60s to 195.5 today."

Stunning, isn't it? It's becoming more and more "normal" to carry excessive body weight . . . and lots of it. But no matter how normal it may seem, or how common it may be, the devastating effects of being overweight are oblivious to the norms. Being 30 pounds overweight, which is common today, is just as bad for your health as it was 50 years ago. Really, due to factors such as the chemical content in "modern" foods and increasing levels of stress, it's probably worse.

Of course, the *average* weight gain has been about 30 pounds. Statistically, though, for every person who has not gained a pound, there is someone who has gained 60. The detriment to our health has been significant. The extra load on the heart alone is devastating. (Imagine having to wear, everywhere you go, a 60-pound flak jacket?)

How can you reach and maintain your proper weight? First, it's helpful to know what your proper weight is. And somewhat ironically, the best way to measure your ideal weight is not with a scale at all, but with a tape measure.

There are simply too many variables to use body weight as an accurate measure of health. For instance, some people are naturally thin, and others are of stocky build. Certain top athletes are measured as overweight by the scale, but they are actually trim and have very low body fat. It's their large muscles that make them heavy. The scale measures them as overweight, but they are not. Furthermore, because stomach weight is the most dangerous weight, your waistline is very key to your health.

Note: To show the folly of using the scale as your main weight-loss measurement: some people who begin an exercise program might gain a few pounds during the first month or two. This may cause them to stop exercising, giving up on it as a failure. The only thing that failed, though, was their understanding of what was really taking place: They may have gained five pounds of muscle and lost two pounds of fat. As far as muscle and fat content go, they have made substantial improvements in both. But if the scale is viewed as the sole measure of success, the program appeared to not succeed. If they had stayed with the program, in no time their muscle gain would have leveled off, but they would continue to lose fat, and the scale would indicate weight loss, and they would look and feel much better.

So what should your waist reading be? The formula is actually very simple. Your waist should not exceed one-half of your height, measured in inches. For example, if a person is five foot ten inches tall (70 inches), their waist should not exceed 35 inches. Please note the chart that follows, which is a guideline to healthy waist measurements:

Waist-Height Chart

If Your Waist is:
Half your height or less: You are in Target Zone
1 to 5 inches over half: Slightly Overweight
5 to 10 inches over: Overweight
10 to 15 inches over: Very Overweight
15 to 22 inches over: Extremely Overweight
> 22 inches over: Extremely Obese

Note: Measure your waist at its largest point, usually near your belly button.

If you are in your target zone, that is excellent. But please note that the ideal measurement is, perhaps, a few inches below the top of the target zone. Getting back to our example of the 5'10" inch person with the 35-inch waist: that person, if they wanted to be in absolutely tip-top shape, would probably do even better at about 31 - 32 inches. If you want to use a figure to measure your figure, the multiple of about .45 is just about perfect. (Your ideal waist measurement should be about 45 percent of your height in inches. Use this formula: Your height in inches x .45 to calculate.)

Please realize that weight loss normally comes at a gradual pace, and so does waist reduction. So plan to lose one inch at a time, or even a fraction of an inch at a time, at the pace that is right for you.

Why are we gaining so much weight? The *Washington Post* article, mentioned at the start of this chapter, identifies the reasons behind the problem: "It basically boils down to three factors: we're eating less healthy food, we're eating more of it, and we're not moving around as much." All three factors are addressed in this book.

Note: Here is one more important and practical reason to remain at or near ideal weight as an adult: Clothing. It is expensive and frustrating to repeatedly have to discard and buy new clothing as our weight fluctuates. Some have had to purchase several additional wardrobes in their lifetimes for the sole reason that their clothing no longer fits.

Have you ever noticed how older gentlemen who are trim sometimes dress in a really dapper style? Very often, they've held to their general weight their entire lives, and thus they can collect a pretty good wardrobe and can afford to buy fine clothing. Additionally, because they are trim, they simply look good in their clothing.

Second Note: Can you spot-lose fat in specific areas, such as your stomach? The answer: No, you can't. While you can build muscles in specific areas, such as exercising those specific muscles, your fat belongs to your entire body and not to that region. That means that your body controls where your fat is burned, and you can't do anything to alter that.

Your fat will generally burn off in the reverse order that it appeared. In other words, if your stomach is your trouble spot and you store fat there first and most, guess where your fat will be the most persistent and burn off last? Yes, your stomach.

Third Note: I mentioned earlier that measuring your waist is more effective than measuring your body weight. And it is.

However, I recommend that you keep your scale handy and check it from time to time. If I lose ten pounds, I want to see it in a big, bright, digital display.

29. Don't Lose Weight to Get Healthy; Get Healthy to Lose Weight

Can you imagine the folly of someone who, when assessing their health, only went by one indicator, perhaps blood sugar? They may think: "As long as my blood sugar is in the healthy range, I'm in good shape."

Not so fast, tunnel-vision dude. Your blood sugar may be healthy, but your blood pressure may be so high that your head is about to take orbit, your pulse jumps sky high at the most minimal effort, your cholesterol is so high that your blood resembles cheese, and your face is glowing red like a rural stop light at midnight.

Most do not make this mistake with regard to blood sugar, but *many* make this mistake with regard to body weight. They believe that as long as their weight is in target range (according to some chart, no doubt), they are healthy.

Body weight is one indicator of your health. But *only one*. Please don't make the mistake of hinging your assessment of your health solely on your body weight.

I'll make a statement now that may surprise you: I'd rather be fifty pounds overweight and otherwise in good health than to be at target weight but otherwise in poor health. You can live a normal, active life while you are fifty pounds overweight, but if you are in poor health, it's almost impossible to live a normal, active life.

Many people believe that if they lose weight, they will be healthy. There's some merit to that. But they are really viewing the equation backwards. It's better to get healthy to lose weight. Why?

As you get healthier, your metabolism gets stronger. This allows you to function better with less food intake—and you'll also have fewer cravings. By eating a more healthful and nutritious diet, and by improving your metabolism, you'll lose weight. But it all starts with eating a healthier diet (and not a dietary trick like an extremely low-carb diet). Add exercise into the equation, and your health will improve even more and your weight will continue to drop as a result.

Remember, you don't just want to lose weight. More importantly, you want to be healthy. By focusing on improved dietary, exercise, and other health building habits, you can get healthier. As you do so, you can lose the weight you want to and look and feel vibrant in the process.

30. Get Adequate Sunlight

"I Got the Sun in the Mornin' (and the Moon at Night)" –
Irving Berlin, Ethel Merman, Betty Hutton, Judy Garland, Doris Day, Dean Martin, et al.

The song title quoted above is from a popular 1946 musical, and it highlights one of the basic needs of the human race (and the entire animal and plant kingdom). Having the "sun in the mornin'" is a great way to start the day.

Actually, you don't have to get your daily dose of sun in the morning. Depending on your circumstances, you can enjoy being in the sunlight at any time of the day. Still, there's nothing like natural morning light for improved health. Why?

Just as the moon controls the oceanic tides, the sun controls our "internal tides," called circadian rhythms. Sunlight signals our body that the day has begun; this has an effect on so many of our body's cycles, hormonal and otherwise. The sun controls our wakefulness as well as our sleepiness. Exposure to the sun gets our internal day-clock ticking, and that pays huge dividends at night when it's time to go to sleep. The body responds and prepares for sleep at some point after the sun has set.

Sunlight helps in other ways, besides supporting our waking and sleep cycles. One important way is that sunlight is an antidepressant. The perils of SAD (seasonal affective disorder) have been thoroughly researched and are widely known. During the winter months, especially in northern areas where the sun shines but is not strong and the days are short (think Alaska), or areas with a persistent cloud cover (think Oregon and Washington), rates of minor blues as well as severe clinical depression can jump.

Furthermore, sun on the skin is a key way for the body to make the all-important vitamin D. Most people have insufficient levels of vitamin D in their blood, but those who spend lots of time in the sun, such as outdoor workers or beachgoers, enjoy healthy levels of vitamin D.

One excellent way to get additional sunlight is to walk every day. Even on cloudy days you'll still benefit, but to a lesser degree, from the natural light. Seattle physician Ralph Golan recommends taking your daily walk without wearing eyeglasses if at all possible and if it is safe for you to do so. The light interacts with the eyes, and glasses can, to some degree, block this effect, especially if they are tinted.

But what if you find it difficult, or impossible, to get sufficient natural sunlight. Is there anything you can do to simulate the effect? Yes, there is. You can use a special light box that is designed to replicate the sun's light.

These lights, often referred to as "happy lights", typically run between $40 and $80 (USD). Most have a built-in timer, which you can typically set for time periods such as 15-30-45-60 minutes. Please, don't ever look directly into the light, but place the box near you, about 18-24 inches away (see your particular box's instructions), and then go about your business, such as eating breakfast near the box or while working at your computer. The better light therapy boxes have a rating of at least 10,000 lux.

You may be wondering if exposure to bright household lights will substitute for the natural sun or a light box. The answer is no, they will not. And here's why: There's much more to the sun's light than just brightness. The sun has a special spectrum of lighting and a distinct wavelength to its light. Light boxes do a good job of replicating the sun's lighting characteristics; regular household lights do not.

Personally, I find nothing more effective than a light box to reset my circadian rhythms and to get into a better sleep pattern.

A Quick Note about Vitamin D Production: The more skin that is exposed to the sun's light, the more vitamin D the body will produce. It's important to know that vitamin D is not produced the moment the sun hits your skin. Rather, the sun interacts with your skin's oils, altering them, and then, during the next 48 hours or so, vitamin D is produced and absorbed from the sun-charged oil on your skin.

That means that you'll benefit very little if you take a shower and wash the oil off your skin soon after your exposure to the sun. If you are trying to boost your vitamin D from the sun, refrain from washing your skin with soap for a while after your exposure. If you do need to shower, perhaps use soap only on key areas of your skin, and allow the oils to remain on other areas, such as, well, un-key areas (arms, legs, etc.) for a time.

The sun, our nearest star, is amazing. We need its light. Be diligent in allowing the sun to have a positive effect on your physical and emotional health.

31. Enjoy Restful Sleep

"Sleep that knits up the raveled sleave of care, The death of each day's life, sore labor's bath, Balm of hurt minds, great nature's second course, Chief nourisher in life's feast." – William Shakespeare

So wrote William Shakespeare in the 1606 play, *Macbeth*. Shakespeare clearly appreciated the benefits of sleep, and 1606 was a time when people got a lot more sleep at night than they do today. (Let's face it, Thomas Edison, Alexander Graham Bell, Henry Ford, and Bill Gates hadn't been born yet, and there was way less to do at night.) Today, many people live with a huge chronic sleep debt, lacking sufficient sleep night after night, and that often causes their health, and their lives, to unravel.

Why is getting sufficient sleep so important?

Sleep has a marvelous and necessary effect on the body and brain. The body needs to do a few things while asleep, and that's essentially to rest, to heal, to cleanse, and to rebuild. The brain needs to do multitudes of things, including rest, process the day's events, and dream about any myriads of things. Sleep is extraordinarily renewing to both the mind and the body, and when sleep is peaceful and restorative, it's a great way to spend one-third of your 24-hour day.

And we are all familiar with the term "beauty sleep." That's not just a line. Sleep is a great cosmetic: a good night's sleep definitely adds to beauty, while being in sleep lack contributes to a haggard appearance.

As late as the 1950s, scientists believed that when we sleep, we are more or less in a dormant, slowed down stage of brain activity. Modern science has proven otherwise. Rather, we cycle through various sleep stages, each with distinct traits, including distinct brain patterns, and a specific purpose. You may find learning about the various sleep stages educational, if not fascinating. I'll provide an overview here.

Note: There are currently two scientific models of the stages of sleep. They are very similar to each other with just one slight variation. One model lists four stages of non-REM sleep, and the other lists only three stages. The two different models are as follows:

Model 1	Model 2
Stage 1	Stage 1
Stage 2	Stage 2
Stage 3	Stage 3
Stage 4	REM
REM	

In one model, there are four stages of non-REM sleep. In the other model, stages three and four are combined and simply designated as "stage 3", with no differential between them. In this chapter, I'll use mostly the 3-stage model.

REM sleep refers to rapid eye movement sleep, where the eyes are darting all over the place under closed eyelids. Non-REM sleep, which are the other stages, refers to sleep where the eyes are still. We tend to cycle in an orderly manner through one stage after the other for a total of about six complete cycles per night. Each cycle takes about eighty minutes.

Let's take a brief look at what happens in your mind and body during each phase of sleep:

Stage One: This is the introductory and lightest stage of sleep, and it occurs when you are in the process of actually falling asleep. Some people are vaguely aware that they are falling asleep during this stage. Stage one sleep produces alpha and theta waves in the brain. Because stage one is such a light stage of sleep, you can easily be awoken. Stage one sleep lasts just a few minutes and it prepares your mind and body for the deeper stages of sleep.

Note: Think of how beneficial it is that we begin our sleep in lighter stage one. For instance, it's a sad fact that there are many drowsy drivers on the road, particularly at night. If a driver nods off in stage one sleep, something, such as a tire running over a reflector that separates the lanes, will likely wake that person up. In the deeper stages of sleep, that wouldn't happen. You can only imagine the increase in serious accidents that would occur if we went directly to the deeper stages of sleep.

Stage Two: This stage is a little bit deeper than stage one. During stage two sleep your brain waves slow down but you'll have sudden increases in brainwave activity, which are called "sleep spindles". Stage two lasts quite a bit longer than stage one, and it serves as a link between light stage one sleep and deep stage three sleep.

Stage Three (and Four): Now were basking in the good stuff! Stage three sleep is the deepest stage of sleep, and the brain is producing predominantly delta waves. During stage three sleep your body essentially becomes limp: there is no eye or muscle activity. If there are, though, nighttime events such as sleep walking or sleep talking, they normally occur during this stage.

Stage three is the most restorative stage of sleep. During stage three sleep, the muscles and tissues rebuild, immune function is boosted, growth and development occur, and the body gathers energy for the demands of the next day.

REM (Rapid Eye Movement) Sleep: For many, REM sleep is the most intriguing. Why? Perhaps because it runs contrary to what scientists believed just a few decades ago . . . they believed that while we were asleep, our minds and bodies essentially went into shutdown mode. But during REM sleep the mind and the body, or at least the mind and the eyes, are all over the place.

Most of our dreams occur during REM sleep, and when the eyes are busy darting around, it's likely that person is "viewing" a dream.

During REM sleep, much activity is taking place in the body. Pulse and blood pressure increase, and breathing becomes rapid and irregular. This is just what you'd expect if that same person were viewing an action-packed movie. (Have you ever wanted to go back to sleep to finish a dream? That's how real our dreams can seem to us.)

During REM sleep, the brain gets quite a workout and yet quite a repair session at the same time. It's busy processing events and data from the previous day or days, and long-term memory is developed and refined.

Please note the chart of a typical night's sleep below. Notice how the deeper stages of sleep dominate the early part of the night's sleep, and REM sleep becomes more prominent toward morning.

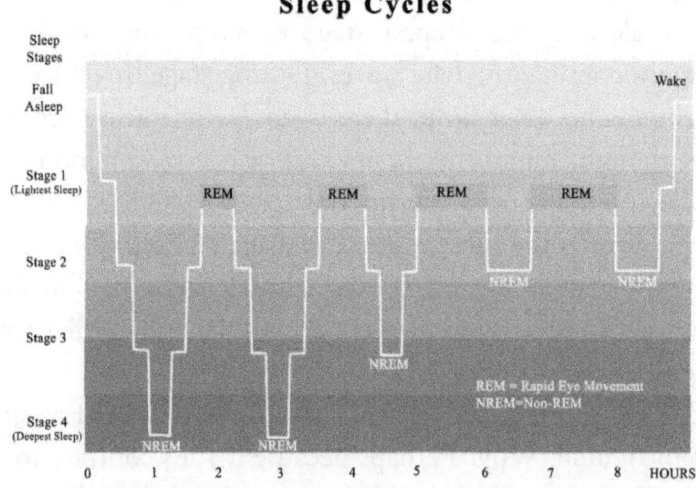

Now that we've enjoyed a basic description of what sleep is and its various stages, I'll discuss sleep a little more and provide some tips that show how to get a good night's sleep every night.

The importance of sleep is often undervalued. But sleep and health are deeply intertwined at many levels. Your need for sleep is just about as important as your need for food, if not more important.

You'll be very hungry after 48 hours without food, but you still may be able to function to a degree and carry out certain tasks. Some people actually feel calm and elated after two days without food. But after 48 hours without sleep, you'd probably be in a state of almost complete disability and in a borderline psychotic condition. (Which, by the way, qualifies you to be an author.)

As important as the proper amount of sleep is, quality is just as important as quantity. If sleep quality is poor, one can awaken from a full night's sleep and still be exhausted and actually feel worse than they did before they fell asleep.

What leads to poor quality sleep? There could be any number of factors . . . anything that stresses the body and mind and keeps the brain or body from relaxing at night will be a detriment to your sleep. One of the most common problems is food, and particularly rich food, that is eaten late at night too close to bedtime. For most of us, burritos and jalapeno peppers washed down with a couple of colas right before retiring will keep the mind and body on high alert all night, and it's almost a certainty that you'd be "fogged in" in the morning.

Here are some tips to getting a good night's sleep virtually every night:

Keep regular sleep hours if possible. Your body functions best when you adhere to certain routines, such as mealtimes and sleep times. Those who sleep at the same time every night are living in harmony with their sleep cycles. They get a little sleepy an hour or so before bedtime, and this sleepiness progresses until, right on schedule, they are ready for their full night's sleep.

Consider establishing a pre-sleep routine. Some find it helpful to turn off communication sources (television, cell phone ringer, etc.) for an hour or so before bedtime. They may read or engage in a gentle conversation. A warm bath or shower helps many to relax.

Many find that keeping the bedroom cool helps them to sleep better. If you've ever tried to sleep in a hot, stuffy room, you know it's not the easiest thing to do.

Most sleep experts recommend that you remove all light sources from your bedroom, including digital clocks. They believe that a complete blackout is best. I'm not sure I agree. After all, we were meant to sleep under the moon's gentle glow in its various stages. Of course, do whatever works best for you.

On the subject of light, make sure to get morning light, even in the form of a light box (happy light), which keeps your circadian and sleep rhythms in a good pattern and strong. Furthermore, research shows that "blue light," which is emitted from such devices as tablets and cell phones, can reduce melatonin output. Melatonin is a hormone that induces sleep, so lowered levels will have a detrimental effect on sleep cycles. It may be best to avoid reading on a device or have exposure to significant light an hour or so before retiring.

Maintain regular mealtimes. Regular mealtimes help keep the circadian sleep rhythms strong. And please, don't eat a large meal within at least a couple of hours before going to bed for the night.

Some people find a "white noise machine" helpful. White noise refers to a steady source of noise, such as from a fan, waterfall, babbling brook, etc. White noise is conducive to sleep, whereas intermittent noise, such as cars and trucks passing, including sirens and horns blowing and screeching brakes, is not. Intermittent noise will definitely affect your brain waves during sleep, leading to poor quality sleep. White noise, which does not affect sleep, can muffle or drown out intermittent noise and contribute to better sleep. We use a Lectrofan in our home, which is a small device that produces fan noise; there are about twenty settings to choose from, and the unit does its job well.

Finally, if you are able to, allow yourself to wake up naturally without the "help" of an alarm clock. It's better to wake up when your body, and especially your mind, are ready to wake up than to be rudely jolted out of a deep sleep or a period of intense dreaming.

Sleep, quality sleep, has a marvelous effect on the mind and body. I used to write cartoons, a few of which have graced/sullied this book. There were times I'd actually wake up with a new cartoon in mind, fully formed, and ready for ink.

I'm not alone in the matter of waking up with a new creation in mind or a problem solved. In fact, I'm in company that is way over my head. Several recording artists have awoken with a new song that they "wrote" during their night's sleep. Both John Lennon and Paul McCartney did this—Paul wrote the songs Yesterday and Let it Be while asleep. (Those two should have teamed up; they may have made something of themselves!) Keith Richards of the Rolling Stones is reported to have awoken in the middle of the night with the riff and words to the hook of "(I Can't Get No) Satisfaction." He recorded them on a cassette and went back to sleep, only to be very pleasantly surprised by what he heard in the morning.

So never underestimate the restorative powers of sleep. Be certain to make quality sleep, in the right quantity, a priority. The benefits to your physical, mental, and emotional health are remarkable.

32. Keep a Regular Routine if Possible

The maverick likes to keep things loose. Sleep? Whenever. Meals? Whenever. Exercise? Whenever; if ever. He doesn't want to be shackled by routines. The maverick, though, is often one sickly fellow.

Research and observation show that the more things we do on a regular schedule as part of a routine, the better. Why is this so?

Regular cycles are built in to the world around us. We know when it's going to be day and when it's going to be night. We know when it's going to be summer and when it's going to be winter. Imagine if we planned a picnic with friends for 1:00 pm on a summer day, but when we arrived, right on schedule, for some reason it was dark as midnight and at the height of a blizzard? That would be quite upsetting, wouldn't it? And yet, that's how your body and mind feel when you keep an erratic schedule. They are never quite sure what's going on.

Just as the sun, moon, and Earth all keep a regular routine—with their sunrise, sunset, moonrise, moon phases, oceanic tides, seasons, and more—so do your internal cycles, known as circadian rhythms. (The word "circadian" is derived from two Latin words: circa [around] and dia [day].) So circadian rhythms are those rhythms that are daily cycles in our bodies. Examples of these are daily fluctuations in your blood pressure, body temperature, melatonin levels, cortisol levels, and more.

One of the funniest scenes I've ever seen on a television program was a lively discussion between Archie Bunker and Mike "Meathead" Stivic about the proper order to put on shoes and socks. Mike was putting on a sock and then a shoe over that sock, and then proceeding to do the same on the other foot. Archie objected, saying that everyone knows that the correct way to do this was to put on both socks first and then both shoes. Then the hilarity began.

That's not what I'm referring to, though, when speaking about keeping a regular routine. Shoes and socks have nothing to do with your circadian rhythms, so if you want to do sock-shoe-sock-shoe, or sock-sock-shoe-shoe, that's up to you. You can even go a little rogue and go shoe-shoe and forget the socks if you like, or you can change the routine whenever you feel like it. But again, it's the circadian rhythms that affect our health.

When those rhythms are consistent, they become strong and ingrained. Those who go to sleep at about the same time every night and wake up at the same time every day can tell you all about it. All of a sudden, at a certain time in the evening, they have no doubt that they'd be a lot happier in bed. And then, right on schedule in the morning, when their cortisol level is just about at peak and their body temperature is low and their pulse is slow, they wake up, refreshed, and they are ready to go for the day.

Those who "play it by ear" have weaker circadian rhythms, and that leads to lower quality sleep, less wakefulness during the day, an erratic appetite, and more.

You have probably experienced the folly of working against your natural rhythms. For instance, have you ever had the following happen to you? You get sleepy at your normal bedtime, but for some reason, you continue to stay up, maybe for two or three more hours. Then, when you finally try to go to sleep, you've stayed up past your natural bedtime and sleep is now elusive. Your body is confused, you are wired, and you just can't fall asleep.

Or have you ever stayed up late with the intention of sleeping later than usual in the morning. But at your normal wake time, your waking cycles have begun, and no matter how late you have stayed up and how tired you are, you just can't stay asleep? When that happens, the rest of your day will not feel very good.

But wait, some may ask, isn't living on a regular schedule boring? Not at all. In fact, quite the opposite is true. Keeping regular routines for eating and sleeping gives you more time and energy. With that time and energy you can be much more adventuresome in your life, much more creative, get a lot more accomplished, and have a whole lot more fun.

Or maybe I should put it this way: If you find living in a state of constant clinical jet lag exciting, go ahead and keep erratic hours and eat at erratic times. Because that is exactly the effect they produce.

What about night workers? Can they live a healthy life? Surely those who must stay up while it is dark and sleep while it is light have a disadvantage, but yes, they can still live a healthy life. How? By following these same principles of keeping a regular schedule. They should have regular times for sleep and for meals. The body will adjust to the circumstances and build the appropriate circadian rhythms.

Of course, as a word of caution: while keeping regular routines is important, there is a need for balance. If a meal is 15 minutes late, or early, it's not the end of the world. Keep a regular schedule, but do so with a reasonable spirit.

There is one more interesting way that keeping a regular routine leads to a better life. It has to do with a concept called *decision fatigue*. This refers to the barrage of decisions all of us have to make every day, which start almost the moment we wake up. After a while, all of those decisions take their toll, and they really do lead to fatigue. This is one of the reasons stores place candy bars and like items next to the cash registers. They figure that by the time you have reached that point, you already have decision fatigue, so if that Snickers bar looks good, you're not even going to think about it anymore . . . you're just going to grab it. (And, it should be noted, that all types of fatigue lead to cravings for sugary-type foods.)

One way to reduce decision fatigue is to automate as many activities as possible. If you have a regular time for bedding down and waking up, and if you have a regular time for meals, it helps reduce decision fatigue.

Noted sage Benjamin Franklin is credited with this well-known saying: "Early to bed and early to rise makes a man healthy, wealthy, and wise." There's truth in that at two levels, one that is obvious and another that is perhaps not. The obvious: Getting to bed early, which is more in harmony with the sun's daily cycle and our body's natural rhythms, is beneficial. The not so obvious: By doing this, by getting to bed early, we'll be keeping a regular routine for our sleep, which will most likely lead to a more regular routine for our meals, both of which will benefit our health significantly.

Keeping a regular routine for things that should be routine is a huge stepping stone to better health.

Note: How many decisions did I have to make while writing and preparing this book? Of course, there's no way to know for sure, but I would estimate that number is close to 250,000, or one quarter of a million. I'm so glad that Microsoft Word automates many more decisions for me, which lets me concentrate on the good stuff.

33. Accept Reality: And Deal With it Wisely

One of the most important lessons any of us can learn in life is to accept reality. Once we do that, we can mobilize our resources to deal with that reality wisely and successfully.

The most classic case, perhaps, is that of the alcoholic. An alcoholic will never begin recovery until they first admit that they have a drinking problem.

Again, that's a classic, or even a stark example. But there are more subtle ways that not accepting reality can interfere with the functioning and successes of our lives. One of my favorite stories involves a Rhodes Scholar, a hall-of-fame professional basketball player, and a United States senator—all wrapped up in one. We're talking none other than Bill Bradley, who studied at Princeton and Oxford, played basketball for the New York Knicks, was elected to the Basketball Hall of Fame, and went on to become the senator of New Jersey and a top presidential candidate.

Mr. Bradley told a story that occurred early in his professional basketball career that sheds light on the matter of accepting reality. He mentioned that at the end of one close game, he made a costly mistake that ultimately caused his team to lose. Bill's mistake stayed with him for several days. He kept replaying it in his mind, chastising himself about it and wondering what would have been if he had not committed the flub.

Guess what happened next? During the next several games, Bill played poorly and committed mistakes, one after the other, and his personal and team's performance suffered.

A kindly veteran teammate saw what was happening, spoke with Bill, and taught him an important lesson. He said: 'Bill, no matter what happens during a game, and no matter what you've done right or wrong, you've got to let it go immediately after the game and begin preparing for the next one. You can't live in the past in this league—you'll get eaten up if you do.'

Bill's focus got stuck on that one game—or really on that one mistake. He could not accept that he made the error, and it was crippling him from moving forward. Bill learned the lesson, took each game one at a time, and, as mentioned, ended up in the Basketball Hall of Fame.

Dieters sometimes have a hard time accepting a certain reality: the fact that they veered from their diets. They may turn one dietary transgression into a long-term stumbling block. How much better to admit the one mistake, learn any necessary lessons, make adjustments to correct it, and then move forward in a positive course. The lesson: it's not beneficial to cry over spilled organic almond milk: clean it up, and move forward—the sooner the better.

If you are in poor health in one way or another, accept that reality, figure out how you got that way, and then take positive steps to repair the problem.

If you need to make any health changes, such as losing weight or getting in better condition, don't view the corrective course as a "punishment." Rather, focus on the good, getting back to the basics, and view those changes as opportunities for a better future.

The point: we all have only so much time and energy. When we accept the reality of our situation, we are now in position to use all of our time and energy in a positive way to overcome our problem.

34. Be Your Own Person: Think for Yourself

"If all of your friends jumped off of a tall building into the street, would you do it too?" – Quote attributed to probably every parent who ever lived, with slight variations.

That opening quote. How many times I heard that as a child! It always came after I did something foolish but defended my actions with the fact that "all the other guys did it."

Looking back, those words were filled with sage wisdom. But I never really appreciated them as a child. It was easier, and way more fun, to go along with the crowd and to hope that I escaped reaping any negative consequences.

And yet, when we grow up, most, perhaps, keep that same mental disposition toward life itself. They reason: "Everyone else is eating junk food filled with chemicals, hormones, and other non-edible matter. Why shouldn't I?" Or it could be: "All the other drivers speed and tailgate, why shouldn't I." It's so easy to ignore the results of the consequences, until they hit us so hard that they floor us, and then it's often too late.

If you want to enjoy better health, and if you want true happiness, it's imperative that you learn to think for yourself. In this world we live in, with its misinformation, greed, and sometimes blatant stupidity (remember the multi-million dollar business Pet Rocks?), doing so is a necessity.

Let's illustrate this with a question: Would you rather navigate a rowboat, a canoe, or a motorboat? There's all types of legitimate answers to that question. Some like the power and speed of a motor, others like the gentle pace and peaceful sounds of the rowboat or canoe. But now let's change the question a little: Would you rather navigate a rowboat, a canoe, or a motorboat in rough seas with high winds, powerful currents, choppy waters, and huge sea creatures, such as sharks and whales? The addendum to that question is pretty much a game changer.

And that's how it is in the world we live in. If we just drift along and go with the flow, we could easily end up where we don't want to be—and in big trouble. Sad to say, today's world has given us very rough conditions. Thinking for ourselves is our motor; it allows us to stay in safe areas and maneuver away from trouble or danger quickly.

One obvious example of this is with diet. So many of us were raised on the typical Western diet: hot dogs, hamburgers, mac and cheese, sodas, apple pie, cakes, cookies, chips, and the like. Some even feel somewhat patriotic about that diet, as though it's somehow un-American not to continue to eat those foods. And they continue to eat them long after they have grown up and are responsible for their own food choices and health decisions.

Has this continued dietary pattern served the public well? A look at the human condition—peoples' body shapes, their complexion, and even their countenance and mood—provides a definitive answer. It's not working in any way, bloated shape, or form.

But yet, those who break out of the mold and have a veggie sandwich with avocado and lime-cashew dressing on whole grain bread are often ostracized as the weird ones. They're not; they are the ones who are thinking for themselves and acting wisely by trying to protect the only body they have. Early disability and early death are not options to them, and they are taking steps to ward off such a possibility. Frankly, those content with remaining on a diet that is slowly disfiguring, poisoning, disabling, and killing them are the ones who could use a good talking to and a wakeup call.

When you think for yourself and you make the effort to properly care for yourself, you are to be applauded, even praised. You're acting with prudency and practical wisdom.

Izabella Wentz, who is a top-notch pharmaceutical physician with a huge web and YouTube presence, refers to these ones admiringly as "health rebels." And so it is . . . if you want to enjoy a healthy life and look like a healthy person, you must rebel against the norms of this system and its horrendous typical diet.

Another way to think for yourself is your view about how others affect your life. While you should care what other people think, and you should try to take their thoughts and feelings into consideration, you should never allow them to cross the line and dictate to you your choices in life or cause you to make decisions that you'll regret. You are the one who has to live with the consequences, not them.

Those who think for themselves are logical people, they are inquisitive people, they are sensible people, they are shrewd people, and they are smart people.

They'll ask such questions as "What's in that dish?" "Who's going to be at that party?" "How long has that chicken salad been sitting out?" "When was that fish delivered to your store?" Even better, when it comes to fish, they'll ask to smell the fish before they buy it. Unless they really, really, trust the store, doing so could save them a ruined meal and a big hassle. (If you think about it, we probably all smell the fish at home before we cook it. That's good, but the most logical time to smell it is before we spend our money on it.)

Thinking for ourselves, stepping outside of the norm, and asking questions might seem like a lot of work. In reality, it's liberating! Taking control of your life gives a feeling of confidence that you could not otherwise experience. Again, it's your powerboat against the turbulence of the world.

In summary, be your own person and think for yourself. By doing this, you will be taking control of your own health and life, and that's a very good thing!

35. Maintain Sound Oral Health

No, this is not a typical chapter about the benefits of maintaining sound oral health where the focus is solely on the teeth and gums. Rather, this discussion will focus on why maintaining sound oral health is beneficial not only to the mouth, but to the health of the entire body.

When someone neglects their oral health, the damage to the mouth is pretty evident. There are more than the usual amounts of nerve pain, fillings, lost teeth, crowns, bridges, implants, and the like.

But now, let's change our viewpoint and look at poor oral health as it affects the entire body and person.

First and foremost, your mouth collects bacteria at a rapid rate. When your breath goes into funk mode, that's a clear indication that your mouth is loaded with harmful bacteria. When your teeth become covered with a rough film, that's an indicator of bacteria too.

When you think about the location of your mouth in relation to your entire digestive system, you can perhaps see the problem. Your mouth is by no means an unattached entity. Rather, what's in your mouth is essentially in your stomach and intestines, because every time you swallow, you are swallowing the contents of your mouth, and even without swallowing, your saliva easily works its way down to the rest of your digestive system. How much better to clean all that goo out of there before it builds up and to keep your mouth fresh. For this reason, it's best to brush your teeth at least twice a day, if not three times a day, if not after every meal.

What about flossing? I can answer this by quoting, from memory, something I saw in a *Reader's Digest* some twenty or thirty years ago. The article was written by a dentist who referred to the space between our teeth as 'cesspools, two rows of cesspools in our mouths; cesspools that could only be cleaned by flossing the teeth on a regular basis.' Um, enough said. Actually, brilliantly said. You don't want cesspools regularly dripping into your digestive system.

What about toothpaste? Is it necessary to use fluoride toothpaste? There are two polar thought processes on this, and I believe that the balanced view is right in the middle of the two. I think that four out of five dentists, or more, would agree.

Fluoride is a chemical, and it can be harmful to the human body. For that reason, some believe that fluoride is to be avoided at all costs, and they will use "natural" toothpaste that is free of any chemicals.

The other view is that fluoride prevents cavities (which has been clinically proven), so our toothpaste should contain fluoride, as should our drinking water.

And now, the middle ground. Yes, fluoride does prevent cavities, but that's only been proven to be the case when fluoride is applied directly to the teeth. Therefore, it makes sense to use a good toothpaste that contains fluoride. But please, make sure to rinse very well after you brush to keep as much fluoride out of your system as possible. (And when you rinse, don't just put some water in your mouth, move it around a little and then spit it out. Rather, use your mouth muscles to create as much force as you comfortably can when swishing. Doing so will force the water through the spaces between your teeth and will otherwise lead to a much more thorough rinse process.) This way, you are allowing fluoride to do its work on your teeth, but you are protecting your liver and cells from this otherwise potentially harmful chemical.

Good dental care brings so many benefits. If you have all of your teeth, you'll chew your food more efficiently. If you don't need extensive dental work, you'll save money that could better be used for higher quality food. If you are conscious of your oral health, you'll probably be less apt to eat sugar, which is a major cause of dental caries and many other health issues.

But most of all, remember that tremendous amounts of bacteria pool in the mouth, which creates a steady stream of percolating bacterial goo going directly into the digestive system. Brush well, brush often, and keep things clean. Your mouth, your entire body, and even your friends, will be appreciative.

36. Have Fun: Immerse Yourself in a Hobby or Something Else You Love

It is clear that human beings thrive on several things. We thrive on love, we thrive on good food, and we thrive on individuality and creativity.

Much of our time is spent in doing things we have to do: work, school, paying bills, shopping, and other obligations. But thankfully, most of us have at least some free time—time to schedule any way we like. What we do with those times is important and can enrich our lives, and it's important to do something we love.

When I was young, I loved to play most sports. Football was my favorite. Every day after school, during football season, the guys would get together and play "pickup games." We'd play for hours, and the time seemed to just fly by. Why? We were having fun, we were with friends, and we were doing something we liked. Personally,

I immersed myself in the mental aspects of the game, trying to figure out strategic ways to win. I'd pay attention to everything, and I'd locate weaknesses and tendencies in the other teams' offenses and defenses. We'd play till dark and then go home. It was so much fun, that we'd occasionally play in snowstorms.

Now I'll move to a grown up experience. Circa the year 2000, I was involved in one of the most interesting projects in my life. I was creating a computerized program that considered and weighed about 20 risk-factors for heart attack and stroke. Based on those factors, the program printed out a risk level of heart attack and stroke as well as instructions for lowering risk. It also calculated life expectancy based on those factors. The program was purchased by a group of doctors in Atlanta.

I had never programmed computers before, so I was fascinated by the process and all of the math and judgment calls involved. One day, while I was working on the program, I decided to cook a baked potato. So I put a potato in the microwave oven and set the timer at 8:00 (eight minutes). I immediately went back to my computer, and, to my irritation, as soon as I sat down the beeper on the microwave began to sound. As I headed back to the kitchen, I guessed that maybe I had mistakenly set the microwave at: 80 (80 seconds) instead of 8:00 (8 minutes).

To my surprise, when I opened the microwave door, the potato was steaming and sizzling. I stuck a fork in it (a real one; not a proverbial one), and sure enough, the potato was fully cooked.

So what happened? I was so immersed in the fun and challenge of making that program that eight minutes seemed like eighty seconds.

Okay, enough about me (for now). This book is about you. And my suggestion is to find one or more activities that you enjoy, and then immerse yourself in them on a regular basis. You are unique. Do what is fun for you. Do what makes you you!

My marvelous grandmother, Becky, loved to do two things: she loved to knit, and she loved to give gifts to her family members. That combination kept her knitting for hours and hours, year after year, and she found much satisfaction in every minute of it. We enjoyed the fruits of her labor of love, and we all had colorful and special sweaters, hats, scarfs, and more.

My dear friend Nathan loves jigsaw puzzles. He can work a puzzle for many hours on end, and he still wants to keep at it. His mind locks onto the joy of what he is doing and dismisses the troubles of the world.

There are so many activities that we could immerse ourselves in: games, sports, reading, playing with the kids or grandkids, playing with our pets, photography, painting, and so on.

If you enjoy television, is that a good source of immersion? Probably not. Passive entertainment, such as merely watching, does not provide the same benefits as active entertainment, where you are involved and accomplishing something.

Sometimes, what you enjoy may come as a complete surprise to others. It may seem out of character. That's fine: if you enjoy it, it's your time. For instance, 1960s football star Rosie Grier, who was a very, very large, strong man, became an aficionado of . . . needlepoint. Mr. Grier became well known as an advocate of his hobby, and he taught needlepoint on television, as well as wrote the 1973 book, *Rosie Greer's Needlepoint for Men*.

Cherish your free time, and use it well. And remember the word "Immerse" in the title of this chapter. Find something you love, and then get lost in it from time to time or even every day. The benefits are outstanding.

37. Laugh Every Day—Maintain a Sense of Humor

Several years ago, my wife and I were vacationing in Naples, Florida. We were at a restaurant, and something got us laughing semi-hysterically. In the process, I strained a muscle near my ribcage. I had to make myself stop laughing, because it hurt to do so. And that rib injury stayed with me for a couple of days. Is that a good memory or a bad memory?

A good memory! Because even though I injured myself while laughing, I'd be a lot more injured if I didn't find reason to laugh, and to laugh often. There's too much stress and nonsense in this world not to find humor and to express that humor in a good laugh. As my dear friend Dr. Ronald Bonahoom sometimes says: "The day I stop laughing is the day I'll start crying."

You will enjoy living more if you look to find humor in everyday life. You will also be healthier, because laughing is known to be a stress reliever and health enhancer.

And learn to laugh at yourself. A person who can't laugh at himself is in serious trouble. You are, in a sense, your most frequent companion. Allow yourself to laugh at yourself when you do something silly.

For instance, I know a story of a man who did something that landed him squarely in the dullard category. Here's what happened: He had just purchased a vehicle that came equipped with hard, clear plastic flaps on the outside of the vehicle that extended down from the top of each window about four inches. He had never seen those flaps before, so he asked the salesperson what they were. The salesperson replied that they were "rain guards." He explained that you can put the windows down when it rains and not get wet.

The first time it rained, the man lowered the windows, and he quickly began to get soaked, so he put the windows back up. He made a mental note to remove those ineffective flaps.

A few days later, he pulled up to the drive-thru window of the local pharmacy. The window attendant mentioned that she had the same make and model vehicle. She asked him how he liked the rain guards. He replied that he didn't like them at all, because they didn't work. She asked what he meant. He said that the first time it rained, he put the windows down and both he and the inside of the door got soaked. She then asked him how far he put the windows down. He said "all the way." She replied that the guards were designed so that the windows should only be lowered to the same distance that the guards extended down the window.

Let me tell you, when the drive-thru attendant said that, did I ever feel stupid! Yes, that was me. I generally take a measure of pride in being able to think logically, and I write Sudoku instruction books, and Sudoku is pure logic. But let's face it, I whiffed majorly on that one.

But to me, that's another good memory. I love that story. First of all, it's a little humbling to realize how silly and thoughtless you can be at times, and there's definitely humor in that story, no matter who the culprit was. I've told that story to an audience of a hundred, and they loved it. So again, find humor where you can, even if you are the generator of the humorous flub.

By the way, laughter is not only a psychological release. It's a physical one too. Laughing releases such positive feel good hormones as endorphins. So laughing is a huge stress reliever.

And a shout-out here to the only two people I know who can make me laugh hysterically: my friend Geoff Aitken, and my wife Rae. Both have literally put me on the floor to the point that I could not stand up anymore. Geoff would say something hilarious, and then he'd fight to hold in his own laughter, especially in a public setting. He'd turn beet red in the process and his whole body would shake and quiver as he tried to keep everything in. That was always enough to get me going. And Rae sometimes starts to laugh so hard that neither of us can stop. We once had to pull off of a major highway because I couldn't see the road anymore. (Note to Misty, My State

Farm Agent: You didn't read that.) The funny things in life tickles those two, and it's pleasingly contagious.

I've been talking-the-talk about humor, but now it's time to walk-the-walk. For your enjoyment, I hope, here are a few of my favorite funny quotes and a cartoon or two that I had a part in creating.

Funny Quotes:

Roger Eschbacher: "The pen is mightier than the sword unless it's a real sword in which case the guy with the pen should run away fast."

Jeff Shaw: "When I was a boy, my mother wore a mood ring. When she was in a good mood it turned blue. In a bad mood, it left a big red mark on my forehead."

Jimmy Carter, about wife Rosalynn: "I've never won an argument with her; and the only times I thought I had I found out the argument wasn't over yet."

And an unknown author: "Irony: the opposite of wrinkly."

Additional Paths to Better Health

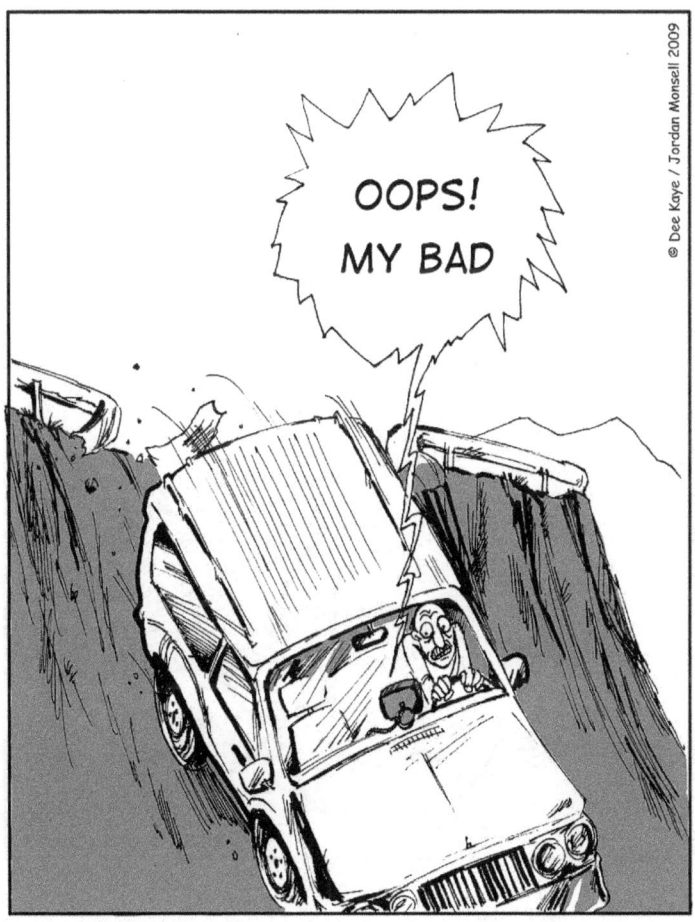

Ed was just beginning to trust his off-brand GPS, and then . . .

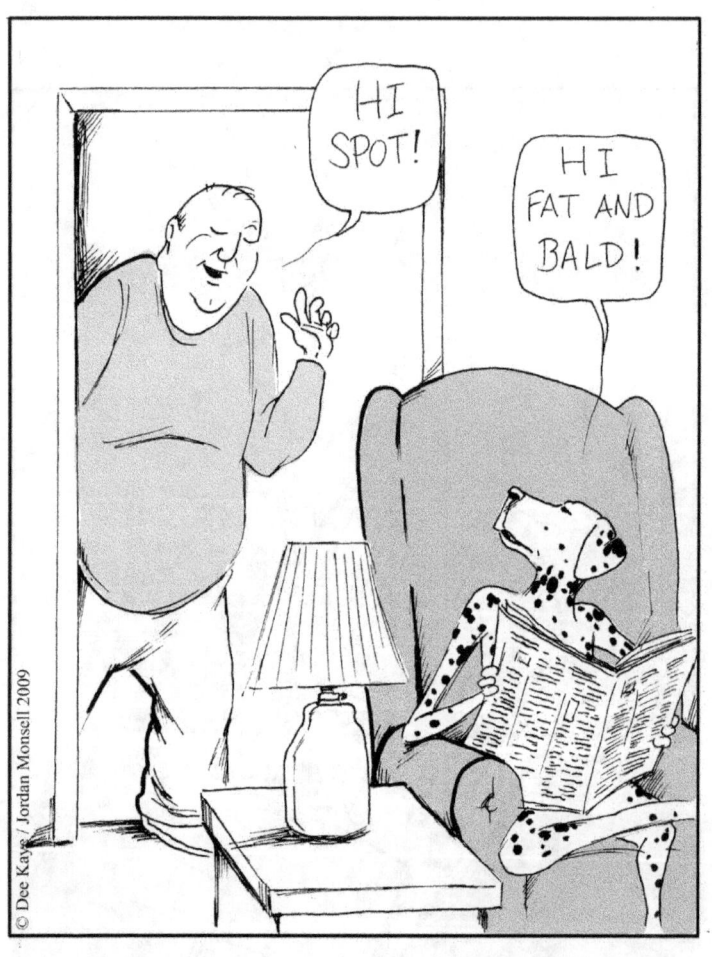

38. Avoid Negative Thinking; Think Positive Thoughts

Positive thinking emboldens. Negative thinking disheartens.

Briefly, I'll share two sports experiences from my past that show how positive or negative thinking can be like a switch that either leads to success or failure.

The first is from my days as a high school high-jumper. A phenomenon happened on several occasions, and it made an impression on me . . . When you jump in competition, you start at a low height, and when you clear that, the bar is raised, usually by an inch or two. That process continues until the event is over.

At the lower heights, the bar looked so easy to clear, and it was. As the bar was raised, it mentally seemed to get *gradually* a little more difficult with each incremental increase. But when I reached the limit of my ability, here's what happened: the next time the bar was raised even an inch, I'd look at it and immediately feel helpless. That bar suddenly looked like an impossible barrier to clear. It was as though it had been raised not an inch, but a mile, like it was resting between two skyscrapers. I knew I didn't stand a chance of clearing it. And then guess what happened when I jumped . . . I missed, but not by an inch. I'd miss by about a foot, even though the bar was only an inch higher. My form was terrible, and I didn't even come close. Why? I knew I was outmatched, and I lost my composure and fell apart. That was the flipped switch of negative thinking, and it rendered me without a chance.

Now, let's see the other example: how the switch of positive thinking was activated. I was never much of a baseball player, but even as a young adult I liked to occasionally stop at a batting cage and hit some baseballs. One day I went to a cage and decided to try the one with the fastest pitching machine. And fast it was. That ball was being flung at about 90 miles per hour. The ball was barely visible, and it made a hissing, smoking sound as it passed me, which it did frequently. I remember feeling some fear, just in case the ball was off course and came toward my head or face—at 90 miles per hour, there's not a lot of time to react and get out of the way. Therefore, I was standing cautiously and swinging tentatively; I was in self-preservation mode.

After a couple of rounds of flailing away (a round was each set of balls the machine threw per coins inserted), I realized how accurate the machine was. Virtually every pitch was in the strike zone, and the ones that weren't were close. I remember saying to myself: "As fast as the ball is, it's not going to hit me. I'm not afraid anymore." At that moment I flipped my mental switch from negative to positive. From that point on I stood with confidence and began whacking the ball all over the cage with authority. Just the change in my thinking made the difference.

That was sports, but the same principle holds true in all facets of life. When we are afraid of failing, or when we think we can't succeed, we are almost assured of failing and not succeeding.

That's not to say that we should have a positive attitude to the point of being unrealistic. The "I can do anything" attitude can get you in trouble. If you are tone deaf, you're not going to be able to become a master orchestra conductor, and if you look like me, you're not going to win any beauty contests. (I'm not making this up: I've verified this fact with some friends.) But there are some things you can do to stack the odds in your favor.

The foremost of these is to learn to prepare well. Benjamin Franklin sagely noted: "By failing to prepare, you are preparing to fail." When we prepare well for what is important to us, we gain confidence, and that confidence breeds a positive attitude. In turn, that positive attitude leads to greater success.

Norman Vincent Peale famously wrote the book *The Power of Positive Thinking*, which became a classic and a huge bestseller when it was published in 1952. Here are a couple of gems from that book, which you may want to give deep consideration to:

"Formulate and stamp indelibly on your mind a mental picture of yourself as succeeding. Hold this picture tenaciously. Never permit it to fade. Your mind will seek to develop the picture... Do not build up obstacles in your imagination."

"The way to happiness: Keep your heart free from hate, your mind from worry. Live simply, expect little, give much. Scatter sunshine, forget self, think of others. Try this for a week and you will be surprised."

Negativity will zap your energy and courage. A positive outlook will boost your energy and courage. Prepare to the best of your ability, and then flip the switch to "yes I can." You may be pleasantly surprised by the results.

39. Build and Maintain a Large Circle of Friends

Aloysius T. McKeever once wonderfully said: "To be without friends is a serious form of poverty." Poverty is not a happy word, and those who have been forced to live in poverty know the cruel, cold, ragged, empty pain that it brings.

Okay, if you Google Mr. McKeever you'll learn that he was not a real person at all, but he was a movie character, and a very loveable one, in the 1947 oddball-comedy film *It Happened on Fifth Avenue*. But McKeever was spot on. Life without friends is a lonely, painful existence. You can live in a major city and be surrounded by millions of people. But if none of them are true friends . . . that's poverty indeed.

While the character Aloysius T. McKeever was fictional, the borough of Roseto, Pennsylvania, is not. (A borough is similar to a town or village.) Let's discuss this small community and the fascinating research of Dr. Stewart Wolf as it relates to close friendships and health.

In 1961, while Dr. Wolf was the head of the Department of Medicine at the University of Oklahoma, a colleague, who had previously practiced medicine in Roseto, Pennsylvania, mentioned that he had never known of anyone in that town under the age of 55 to have heart trouble.

Wolf was intrigued, so he assembled a research team to study the people of Roseto, attempting to discover what protected them from developing heart disease.

A thorough examination of the population revealed some interesting findings: the people of Roseto had mostly normal risk factors. Their exercise and smoking habits were similar to other communities, and they were actually more obese and ate more animal fat then the norm. But their rate of death by heart attack was unusually low. What caused this low rate of heart disease?

Here's what the research team concluded . . . the townspeople were protected from stress because they enjoyed an unusually close bond of friendship with family, friends, and neighbors. Roseto was truly a place out of the past, where people knew each other, supported each other, befriended each other, and loved each other.

Stress is a major health destroyer, and when you are immersed in a warm and loving community, your stress levels will lower, as will your risk of heart disease and other illnesses, such as high blood pressure, diabetes, emotional illnesses, and the like. Those warm relationships act as a barrier against major diseases and the damage they cause.

While Dr. Wolf's study and conclusion was considered novel at that time, his work is now accepted by the medical community. University of Maryland psychologist James J. Lynch, in his book *The Broken Heart: The Medical Consequences of Loneliness*, said Wolf's work and similar studies showed social and psychological stresses "may be the most important of all risk factors" in heart disease.

So are you thinking of moving to Roseto to experience such health benefits? Don't bother. Because while the borough of Roseto still exists, the lifestyle that promoted exceptional health benefits does not. In the last fifty-plus years, Roseto has "caught up to the rest of the world" in ways of social values and modern living, and in the process it lost much of what made it different. The health of Roseto residents is now no different than other communities.

Does this mean all is hopeless, that there's no community where you can find this wonderful health benefit? Not at all. In your own personal life you can create such as circle of friends and community no matter where you live.

How do you gain friends? By being a friend. Take an interest in people. Show them you care. Tell them you care. And then back it up. Be there when they need you. Spend time getting to know each other. Stay in touch. Give little gifts that say "I'm thinking of you, you are important to me."

Remember: if you have one true friend, you have a jewel. If you have several true friends, you have a treasure chest. And if you have a treasure chest, you're rich. Never take that for granted and never stop cultivating that treasure chest. Living this way is a huge stress reliever and health builder.

And periodically thank your circle of friends for being your circle of friends, just like I'm about to do . . . You all mean so much to me, and you enrich my and Rae's lives tremendously. Thank you so much! You are a valuable and precious treasure, and we cherish you.

40. Don't Be a Perfectionist, Be Reasonable

According to Darryl Stewart Wellness: "Perfectionism sucks the air out of your uniqueness and leaves you empty, away from who you could become." Sounds like fun, doesn't it?

No, it doesn't. Best-selling author Anne Wilson Schaef adds: "Perfectionism is self-abuse of the highest order." Being a perfectionist will make you, and everyone around you, miserable. In time, though, there won't be many people around you—they've likely fled to protect their own mental health.

What causes one to want to be a perfectionist? Brené Brown, in her book *The Gifts of Imperfection: Let Go of Who You Think You're Supposed to Be and Embrace Who You Are*, explains: "Perfectionism is a self-destructive and addictive belief system that fuels this primary thought: If I look perfect, and do everything perfectly, I can avoid or minimize the painful feelings of shame, judgment, and blame."

Brown herself responds to this thought process by stating: "Perfectionism is not a way to avoid shame. Perfectionism is a form of shame." There is nothing good or glorified about perfectionism.

Perfectionists often have an "all-or-nothing" mentality. That is, if they feel that they can't completely master something, or do it perfectly, then it's not worth doing. This thinking can be very harmful.

As an example, suppose a person has gained some extra pounds through the years, and they know that it would be prudent to lose some weight. Perhaps they decided with their physician that twenty-five pounds was a good weight-loss goal. How might the perfectionist proceed? He might decide that those twenty-five pounds need to be gone in a couple of months, and he then sets that as an unrealistic deadline. Then, after two months, he may have lost only five pounds, which is actually a commendable loss of weight in those two months. But because he didn't reach his goal, he might give up the mission as lost. What happens next?

He may stop trying and return to his old habits and gain those five pounds back the next month with a "bonus" of five more. How sad that would be, but it is a perfectionist trait—all or nothing. Now he is heftier than he was to begin with and is stuck with a bigger problem than he had in the first place. If he had a reasonable goal and stuck with it, eventually he would be at his target weight.

The great artists of the world were probably all diligent hard workers, but they were not necessarily perfectionists. I love this story about the famed composer Chopin, as told by my friend, blind concert pianist Don Lardie. Don mentioned that following a piano concert Chopin performed, a woman approached him and enthusiastically said: 'Your concert was amazing. You were spectacular, and you did not miss one single note.' Chopin replied: 'My lady, I could have played a whole separate concert with all the notes I missed tonight.' Skill, even brilliance, can shine through the restraints of imperfection.

So be the best you that you can reasonably be, do the best that you possibly can do, and then let it go at that. Insist on quality, even excellence, but don't cross the line of expecting perfection. And remember, when you fall short or mess up, it's perfectly okay to laugh at yourself. Doing so takes most of the sting out of the experience. Allow yourself that pleasure!

If you are careful to avoid perfectionist thinking, you won't miss out on the good (albeit imperfect) part of life.

As a PS to this section . . . there are probably a few mistakes in this book, such as typos and grammatical boo-boos. (Most books have them, even after they've been combed through by editors and proofreaders.) I'm not thrilled about that ~~possibility~~ probability, but that's not going to dampen my joy of releasing what I believe is a fine guide to better health.

41. Be Alert to Whatever May Drain Your Energy and Well-Being

There are things out there, way too numerous to mention, that might be draining your health and zapping your energy. So *be alert* to anything that seems to have a negative effect on your feeling of well-being.

I'll share an example from my own personal experience: I tend to get cold easily, and a logical solution seemed to be to use an electric blanket on my bed.

Near the year 2008, here's what happened: I decided to use an electric blanket during the winter to stay warm at night. Before I did, I remembered that I had tried an electric blanket once many years before that, but I stopped using it very quickly. There was something about it I did not like, but I could not remember what that was.

It took me only one night to remember why I stopped using the electric blanket years earlier: I woke up depressed, very depressed, and I stayed that way all day and into the next day.

When I say depressed, I mean that I was physically depressed. I just felt drained and awful. Of course, such a physical condition will be accompanied by mental and emotional depression too. In those ways, I was numb, and there was no way out of it until the physical symptoms wore off.

A little research showed that I was by no means the only one who suffers such a reaction to electric blankets or to electric fields in general.

A friend lived, for a short time, in a home that was almost directly under some rather major power lines. He hated being home, and I loved his description of how those lines made him feel. He said: "It makes me feel weird." That's not exactly a medical textbook description, but I totally got it; I've been there.

To wrap this story up, I bought a gauss meter, which checks three types of invisible fields: Electric, Magnetic, and Radio/Microwave. I don't seem to be affected by high levels of magnetic or radio waves, but when the electric field is high, look out. And electric blankets are off the charts on electric field activity. The fact that the blanket is touching and covering the entire body makes the problem worse.

I'm actually glad that my reaction to the electric blanket was so drastic. If, perhaps, it was less noticeable, I may have used that blanket for years, barely noticing that my energy resources were being continually drained. And even if I did notice, I may not have been able to identify the problem at a lower level of discomfort. My reaction to the electric blanket was as subtle as a sledgehammer, and there was no doubt as to the source of the problem.

There are many common sources of distress, such as food allergies, mold, certain perfumes, cleaning agents, or even a toxic friend or relative. Know your body (and your friends), and pay attention to what seems to be affecting you.

While you should be alert, please don't become a fanatic. Unless you have a very severe allergy or reaction, such as some people do to peanuts, which can be life threatening, be alert, but don't let over-vigilance be an energy drain in itself to you.

Another dear friend of mine, Grant Payne, used to say that 'we are not wired for the stresses we have to deal with.' And he's right. A little stress here, a big stress there, a few moderate stresses here and there, and our bodies and minds begin to suffer fatigue and to break down. With a reasonable spirit, try to minimize the stresses you have on your body and mind. The result can be liberating.

42. Don't Be a Health Food Store Junk Food Junkie

Say what?

This might seem like a strange concept, but there are people who frequent health food stores who are, in effect, health food store junk food eaters. How so?

They go to health food stores but they shop on the fringes, never buying truly healthy foods. That's not to say health food stores typically carry the types of foods that are served in most fast food restaurants, loaded with deep fried fats and white flour and white sugar.

But health food stores carry many foods that are not healthy. While those foods are better than the alternatives found in regular supermarkets, they are not truly health-building foods. (Before we go further, please don't view this as a knock of health food stores. It is not. I love health food stores. They are fun to shop in and they are packed with excellent, health-building foods that you can't find anywhere else. However, not all foods in health food stores are health-building in the true sense of the word.)

I'm speaking from experience, because for years, this is how I shopped in health food stores: I'd go straight for the "protein bars," sodas, flavored (and sweetened) yogurts and kefirs, chocolates, sweetened carob chips, frozen dinners, and the like. It was great for the psyche: I'd walk out knowing I'd invested heavily in "health foods." But it wasn't so good for the body: those foods are not true health builders.

"Protein bars" are usually overloaded with sugars. Health food sodas are sweetened with sugars that may be better than pure white sugar or high-fructose corn syrup, but too much sugar, in any form, is horrible for the body. The sodas in health food stores typically contain as much sugars as regular sodas. Flavored yogurts and kefirs are also typically loaded with sugars, and frozen macaroni and cheese, even if it's sold in a health food store, is still macaroni and cheese. The pasta may be a higher grade, and the cheese may be too, but it can hardly pass as a true health food.

You may have noticed that a common thread of most of these foods is that they contain too much sugar. That's a trick of the health food industry. It goes as follows: Manufacture and sell delicious items that appear to be healthy, but they taste good because they are loaded with sugar. But the sugars used are considered "healthy sugars," because they may be made from fruit (fructose) or honey. Regardless, too much sugar is too much sugar, and it leads to serious health problems such as obesity, diabetes, and heart disease.

Another trick is to label a food "free," and while it's free of some undesirable items, it may be loaded with others. As an extreme example, if a seller of white sugar wanted to, they could write in big bold letters on the box: Fat Free, Cholesterol Free, Gluten Free, BPA free, Dairy Free, and so on.

In the 1990s, low-fat hysteria hit hard. Many believed that a low-fat diet was the way to a slimmer, healthier body. Because of that, many companies began to market low-fat snacks, such as cookies. They tasted pretty good too. Why? Because they were loaded with sugar. Excess sugar made up for the taste and texture that was lacking from the missing fat. And sadly, the effect was the opposite of what the consumer hoped for. Eating sugar puts on more body fat than eating dietary fat, so the bottom ~~line~~ was to gain weight.

So to the question of "are they out to get you?" Yes, they are. Or at least, they have targeted your dollars and they know how to get those. You and your health could easily get caught in the crosshairs.

Remember, it's not the type of store that counts, it's the foods. <u>You are better off going to your local grocery store and filling your cart with healthful foods than you are going to a health food store and buying bars, sodas, candies, ice creams, sweetened yogurts, and the like.</u>

That doesn't mean that health food stores don't have their place. They do, and I've always loved shopping at health food stores. Just make sure you are not using your health food store mainly as a healthier substitute for junk foods.

And in all fairness, in recent years, the health food industry has made an effort to make these foods healthier than in the past. There are now some protein bars with moderate amounts of carbohydrates, some sodas are made with sweeteners like stevia, and Greek yogurts now contain a more moderate amount of sugar.

Quality health food stores have lots of excellent items that will improve your health. And I've always found shopping in health food stores to be a lot of fun. I highly recommend them, but focus on what are truly health-building foods, such as the organic produce, the probiotic foods, the whole grains, seeds, and nuts, the top-of-the-line supplements, the herbs, the fresh juices and smoothies, the fresh-baked breads, Alyssa's Healthy Oatmeal Bites (I had to sneak in a personal favorite), and so on.

43. Be Peaceful

The following few chapters discuss such qualities as being peaceful, forgiving, thankful, generous, and loving. What do being peaceful, forgiving, thankful, generous, and loving have to do with diet and health? A lot, because they are all intertwined with your health and ultimately your diet too. Let's take a look at these qualities as they relate to health.

Peaceful. If we are peaceful in our relationships with others, our minds will be calmer and more at peace. And when our minds are calmer and more at peace, so are our hearts, nerves, and stomachs. Meals will be more pleasant, you'll probably eat more slowly, and your food will be digested much better. Thus, you'll reap more benefits—and less distress—from your diet.

While it's good to be peaceful, it's even more beneficial to be a peace seeker or peacemaker. Look for ways to resolve situations that may arise, perhaps even choosing to let things go that are not really serious. Some like to fight every little thing because, they say, it's the principle involved. But there's also the principle that humans should live peaceful, happy, and healthy lives. Not making issues of smaller things is a smart way to accomplish that.

And please, don't ruin your own peace with unrealistic expectations. When you've done the best you reasonably can, it's fine to feel a sense of satisfaction from your efforts. Let yourself relax and enjoy life. If you've done your best, you deserve to be at peace with yourself.

44. Don't Blow Your Lid

For a time, especially beginning in the 1960s and '70s, psychologists taught that venting one's anger was a good, healthful idea. They recommended periodically letting go of self-restraint and blowing off steam. Their thinking was that as pressure builds up, it's unhealthy for a person to remain in that pressurized state, so venting anger in frustration, perhaps in a good argument, would release that pressure and restore a peaceful condition. Good idea?

Bad idea. You are not a kettle, you are a human being, and you interact with other human beings. There are better ways to deal with stress than mini- or maxi-explosions. Let's look at the reasonableness of this.

Back to the illustration of the kettle: When kettles blow, they emit steam, which is vaporous water. That's not much of a problem. But when human tempers blow, lots of messy and ugly stuff tends to come out, and cleaning up that mess can be difficult or even impossible.

We tend to say way too much when we let loose, and if our words cause pain in the target of our venting, it's likely that painful words may be headed back in our direction. Chances are good that someone is going to get injured, and the damage may linger. Just as someone is likely to get injured when there is physical violence, someone is likely to get injured when there is verbal violence.

Psychiatric and social experts now teach that the intended goal of such a release backfires. Research has proven that those who vent are more likely to do so in the future, and repeatedly, than those who exercise self-control. As David McRaney puts it in his book *You Are Not So Smart*, "Venting *increases* aggressive behavior over time." Thus, the problem gets multiplied. The person who vents remains angry.

What's the best approach? Stay in control, communicate, and get to the source or root of the problem. A good, productive conversation will release much more pressure than a blow-up, and there's no wounds to bind and no mess to clean up. Rather, you've already taken a step in the right direction toward the resolution of the problem.

When you are upset and things seem to be escalating out of control, it might be a good idea to "take your leave." This may involve physically leaving the situation for a time, or simply making a decision to cool down for a bit before delving into the matter.

During this time, put yourself in the other person's place. Try to see it from their point of view. When we do this, we are more apt to realize that we may have had some part in creating the stressful situation. Even if we haven't, we'll still be better able to come up with and implement a solution in a calm and level-headed manner.

And for you tough guys (and gals) out there, exercising restraint and remaining mild-tempered is not a sign of weakness . . . quite the opposite is true: it's a sign of great strength.

45. Be Forgiving

Hanging on to resentment is, simply put, awful for your health. It's been wisely said that holding resentment inside is the equivalent of drinking poison and then waiting for the person you are angry at to die. When you hold on to resentment, you <u>may</u> or <u>may not</u> injure the other person, but you <u>always</u> injure yourself. The major damage is always to you. Resentment will have a negative effect on your stress levels, your disposition, your relationships with family and friends, your blood pressure levels, your pulse rate, your digestion, your sleep, probably your diet, your face (yes, really), and many other important aspects of life.

It's good to remember that all of us make mistakes, including ourselves. How many times have we needed someone's forgiveness? The pressures of life and inborn imperfections make us prone to act selfishly at times. And then there are misunderstandings, which are common in all relationships.

It's been said that "marriage is the union of two good forgivers." That same principle applies to all friendships. If you are reasonable and forgiving, you'll have more friends, and that in itself is a huge stress reliever that will benefit your health. So when you can . . . let it go. It's to your benefit.

46. Be Thankful

A classic example of one who is not thankful is a spoiled child who thinks that the world owes him anything he wants and that everything revolves around him. The child is thankful for nothing (because, remember, it's owed to him), and he is definitely of ill temper and manner and may even throw tantrums when he doesn't get his way. You may have noticed that spoiled children are never happy children.

And this brings us to adults. Some of us never fully grow out of the childish mold just mentioned. We may not literally jump up and down and throw things when we don't get our way, but we find other creative ways to pout and make ourselves miserable.

Learning to be thankful for what we have, and maintaining reasonable expectations of others, is a great way to keep our peace and to take greater pleasure in what we have, including our food and meals. That leads, of course, to better health physically, mentally, and emotionally.

And while it's good to be thankful at heart, it's even better to express those thanks in word and deed. When we thank others, it makes both them and ourselves feel good, and that builds a feedback loop of goodwill and good feeling. Thankfulness leads to a happier, healthier life.

Let's end with a pair of superb quotes from Minnesota-based self-help author Melody Beattie:

"Gratitude makes sense of our past, brings peace for today, and creates a vision for tomorrow."

"Gratitude unlocks the fullness of life. It turns what we have into enough, and more. It turns denial into acceptance, chaos to order, confusion to clarity. It can turn a meal into a feast, a house into a home, a stranger into a friend."

Those quotes are so meaningful and deep that I wish I had written them myself. Actually, I did . . . but I had to use quotation marks to make it legal!

Very well said indeed, Ms. Beattie!

47. Be Generous

A very wise person one said that there is more happiness in giving than there is in receiving. Being generous is a wonderful way to live. The generous person cares about others and looks for ways to help them or to lighten their load. Such a giving spirit is usually returned to us by others. (But please don't fall into the trap of believing that everyone we show generosity to will be properly appreciative of our kind acts. In today's world, sadly, that's not going to happen.) Many mental health experts recommend generosity as a way to increase your own personal happiness, not to mention the positive effect on the recipients of our kindness.

And remember, there are many ways to be generous. One obvious way is with material resources and gifts. But there are other ways of displaying generosity: giving of our time, our energy, our affection, even just our warm smiles—these are all forms of generosity that pay dividends. If we are generous, we'll feel better about ourselves and sleep better. That means better health and more energy.

One of my favorite stories about generosity caught my attention in 1999, and some 20 years later I haven't forgotten it. It involves a man named Robert Thompson. Mr. Thompson was almost penniless when he began a paving company in Michigan some forty years earlier. He worked long, hard hours to make a success of his business. And a success it was. When he retired in 1999, his was the largest asphalt-paving business in the state.

But what Mr. Thompson did when he sold his business and went into retirement makes this story remarkable. A foreign firm bought the business for 422 million dollars. Mr. Thompson deeply appreciated his staff, who he knew was largely responsible for his success. It was widely known that Thompson expected a lot out of his workers, but he was always appreciative and fair in his dealings with them.

On Thompson's final day of work, he had arranged for a company gathering to thank his employees and to say goodbye. But the good stuff was just about to happen . . .

At the end of the event Mr. Thompson handed each employee a letter. He requested that no one open the letter until they returned home.

When they did return home, they were shocked by what they found. They each received a very nice letter telling them how much they were appreciated and how valuable they were as employees. They were also told that it was arranged for them to keep their jobs under the new ownership. That was very generous of Mr. Thompson. But you can probably guess that I'm leaving something out . . . There was a check in each envelope. The eighty workers with the most seniority each received a gift of a minimum of one million dollars. Some key workers were awarded two million dollars.

One man opened the envelope the moment he returned home, while he was still sitting in his vehicle in his garage. He said that he could do nothing more but sit there and weep uncontrollably before he went inside and shared the news with his wife. Instant life change.

Thompson and his wife Ellen, a former school teacher, were not done yet. A few years later they donated 200 million dollars to the embattled Detroit school district to build charter schools. And they've given several large gifts and created generous funds along the way.

Do you need to give millions of dollars to experience the joy of generosity? No. The Thompsons gave of what they had, and we can all do the same. We all have something to share with others, even if that something is a kind word and a warm smile. Generosity breeds good feelings, it increases joy, it makes life better, and it's a health booster extraordinaire.

48. Be Loving

Love is the pinnacle of good qualities. Work hard to develop a loving disposition. This includes kind acts, but it also includes how we view others. Do we tend to focus on their weaknesses and mistakes, or do we focus on their good qualities? Are we patient, or are we quick to take offense? The loving person looks for the best in every person and every situation. They then try to achieve the best outcome possible.

And don't neglect to be loving to yourself. It would be unloving to expect more of yourself then you are *realistically* capable of doing. At the same time, don't set your standards so low that you lack satisfaction in your accomplishments.

And please, never beat yourself up mentally and emotionally. It's exhausting and injurious. It's actually doubly exhausting and doubly injurious. How so?

If you think about it, when someone gets beaten up, it's exhausting to them, and they are often injured. And the person doing the beating gets exhausted and is sometimes injured as well. So if a person beats themselves up, they are assuming both roles, that of the beater and that of the beaten. That's often double the pain, double the injury, and double the exhaustion. Learn to be understanding and kind to yourself, but at the same time reasonable, with realistic expectations. Having this point of view will pay great dividends to your health.

As humans, love is our number one need. It's impossible to be truly happy without being loved and without loving others. Work hard at being a loving, caring individual. If you do, not only will your health get a boost, but your entire life experience will bloom.

49. Don't Ignore the Whispers (Listen to Your Body)

In the 1980s, I had the privilege of being the client of one of the best doctors I've ever known. His name is Rob Krakovitz, and he has a brilliant mind for nutrition and the human body. He was way ahead of his time in the field of natural medicine.

Dr. Rob was known to say: "If you ignore the whispers, you'll soon be dealing with the screams." This succinctly sums up the wise person's attitude toward their own health. If there are whispers—minor pain, discoloration, fatigue, weight gain, sleep issues, and so forth—and if those whispers are ignored, most often they will not just simply go away. They'll get louder and louder until those whispers become screams, and screams can't be ignored.

Visualize this with a dental cavity. If someone notices a dark mark (cavity) on a tooth, but there is no pain associated with that cavity, they have one of two choices. They can ignore the cavity, or they can get it filled. Getting the cavity filled is a minor and relatively painless and inexpensive procedure. But if they ignore the cavity, it won't be long before the cavity spreads to the root and causes intense nerve pain. (If you've never had tooth nerve pain, I'd describe it as someone hammering a nail into your jaw!) At that point, the only options are a root canal or extraction. That's way more painful, invasive, and expensive, than having had that tooth filled. The matter has progressed from whisper stage to screaming.

Does that mean that you need to run to the doctor every time you hear a "whisper"? No. Sometimes, it's good to observe that whisper for a short while. For instance, you may notice a red mark on your skin. You don't recall seeing it before. It's probably best to keep an eye on it for a few days. If it remains, or if it gets worse, it would be prudent to have a physician look at it. But if it fades and disappears, then it was likely just a scratch or nick and nothing to be concerned about.

One of the worst frustrations you can deal with is this: "I knew I had a problem. Why didn't I do something about it before it became a severe medical issue?" Spare yourself of that painful self-blame and a possible catastrophe: pay attention to your whispers, and then act on them if they persist.

50. Take Time For Yourself Every Day

Modern life is often referred to as a "rat race," and for good reason. There are likely huge demands on your time and energy, and it all may seem overwhelming. You may feel as though you are living on a treadmill: always moving and exerting, but never really getting anywhere.

But it's imperative that you take a little time for yourself—or more than a little—every day if possible, and step off that treadmill. Why?

You are unique. No one else is you. But if you don't take time for yourself, you'll never really discover who you are. Find out who you are, and then nurture that exquisite person. Doing so resets you; it grounds you. It helps you keep the sense of who you are. And it helps you to enjoy life and endure its hardships.

To accomplish this, there are so many things that you can do. But there is no one-size-fits-all formula. You must do what you enjoy, what refreshes you, what intrigues you, and what centers you. It can be a hobby, a project, reading, playing with a pet or the kids or grandkids, or even something as simple as spending time outside and noticing the world around you.

I often sit in our yard and take in the surroundings. A few days before writing this section, I sat outside during the day for just about five minutes. In that short amount of time, Opie, the neighbor's adorable cat, came over to visit. I also noticed the cool, fragrant air, the blue sky and white clouds, the dazzling pine trees, the gentle breeze, and the sounds of birds singing and children playing. It was almost like an instant reset. Timewise, enjoying all of that in just five minutes was lots of bang for the buck.

Sitting out at nighttime can have a similar, but different, effect. When you look at the moon, the planets, and the stars, and you think about the huge, huge distance between them—in some cases millions of light years—the effect can be humbling, awe-inspiring, and confidence building. Suddenly, perhaps, your own problems don't seem so monumental after all. As you think about the orderly and precise manner that the Earth is orbiting the sun, once a year, and is spinning on its axis, once a day, and that the moon is orbiting the Earth at the same time, all with precision clockwork, there is a feeling of awe, peace, and serenity.

Taking time for yourself everyday helps you to claim a little of each day as your own. It puts things in perspective, and it reminds us that life is more than just a daily grind. It gets our mind off of our problems and eases our stresses.

It should be noted that taking time for ourselves, especially when we are involved in wholesome activities, not only affects us mentally and emotionally, but also physically. Studies have shown that peace, rest, pleasant activities, and being in nature will almost immediately lower our blood levels of cortisol, the stress hormone. Excess cortisol damages the body in many ways, increasing risk of illness and serious medical issues. That little bit of time we buy out each day, just for ourselves, can significantly lower our risk and enhance our well-being. By all means, carve out some "you time." You not only need it, you deserve it.

51. Stay Educated About Health and Nutrition

One of the best ways to eat a healthy diet and to get and remain healthy is to read about healthy diets and to read about health in general. There are two main reasons:

a. **When you read about health and healthy dieting, you are educating (and arming) yourself.** If you choose your reading material wisely, and you read with discernment, you'll be consistently learning more about the principles and logic of good nutrition and healthful living. Armed with that knowledge, you can make better choices. I'm pleased to report that there is now an abundance of excellent publications that teach principles of sound health. That wasn't always the case. When choosing reading material, avoid fad-like material and focus on what are sound principles of health and nutrition, ones that are backed by logic and that work in harmony with the body's natural cycles and rhythms.

b. **Reading about health is very motivating.** It's amazing how just a few minutes with a good health book can cause a person to change their diet, their exercise routines, and so forth. When you need a good health boost, read about healthy living. It's very motivating, and you'll likely soon be on a better path.

Of course, there is a need to be selective about what you read, because there's a lot of misinformation out there . . . Wonder Bread did not really build bodies 12 ways, Wheaties may be the "Breakfast of Champions," but is it really the breakfast of champions, literally? Some of the old food pyramids were absurd. My home economics teacher in high school told our class that ice cream is the perfect food, because it contains everything important: dairy, protein, fats, carbohydrates, calcium, and often fruit. I'd imagine that her children had quite the fun childhood and quite a rough go of it as adults. And Wiley Brooks, leader of the Breatherian movement, which claims we can get all the nutrients we need just from the air we breathe, was caught, at the height of popularity of the movement, well, you guessed it, sneaking out for a late-night binge on junk food.

So when you select your reading material, look for those sources that offer a balanced approach to nutrition. Specifically, does the diet seem to be in harmony with the way our bodies are designed? If not, it's best to look elsewhere.

Kindle books have changed the way we can shop for our reading material. You can download a sample of almost any book. Look through the sample, and if you find that the book is to your liking and can benefit you in your quest for better health, then you can buy the book on Kindle, which is usually less expensive than the paperback versions.

Sir Francis Bacon once famously said: "Knowledge is power." Through reasonable knowledge, you can own the power to take control of your own health and to make wise health decisions and lifestyle choices. Surely, time spent on reasonable amounts of education regarding your health is well worth it and can reward you with huge dividends.

52. View Your Health Like a Bank Account

Your health can be likened to a bank account that has been given to you—one that was padded with a sizable wad of money when you first received it. For most of us, that's how we started out as children: with reasonably good health and lots and lots of energy. Some of that energy will wane as we progress through the adult years, but it is the course of wisdom to preserve as much of our health and energy sources as we can. How can we do that?

Should you hoard your energy and never use it to work or play? No. Just as a wealthy person would be a fool to never enjoy the fruitage of any of the wealth they have amassed, we'd be remiss to not enjoy a measure of the energy we have.

Notice, please, these two major principles of banking, and see how they relate to health:

1. Don't spend more money than you have in your account.
2. Maintain a program that allows you to continually add to your savings account on a regular basis.

Do you see the correlation to health? If we use more energy than we have, our systems will go "bankrupt". "Bankrupt" is not a pleasant word. Whether it be in reference to our finances or our health, it does not feel very good and it causes a lot of long-term problems.

Therefore, it's important that you add to your health resource account continually. How do you do that? By adhering to the healthful practices discussed in this book. As you sleep deeply each night, eat nourishing foods, get reasonable amounts of mental and physical exercise, maintain a positive attitude, generously treat others with love, and use humor in your everyday life, you'll be building health reserves that will last a lifetime. May you be a health gazillionaire, and may you remain that way for a long, long, time.

53. Smile and Maintain a Happy Disposition

"Keep on smilin', keep on smilin' baby, and the whole world smiles with you." – Louis Armstrong

Entertainer Louis Armstrong, known for his own dazzling smile, was spot on when he sang about the contagious effects of a smile. When people smile, or when they see others smile, it brightens their entire mood. Why is this so?

There are several reasons, both social and physical.

Notice the words of Harvard-educated psychologist Betty Phillips: "Smiling releases pleasure hormones called endorphins, natural painkillers and antidepressant hormones such as serotonin. Smiling reduces stress and boosts your immune system. You can even measure this response quickly with your blood pressure monitor."

And here's a fascinating passage about the power of a smile from an excerpt of a wonderful article by NBC writer Nicole Spector:

"Smiling can trick your brain into believing you're happy which can then spur actual feelings of happiness. But it doesn't end there. Dr. Murray Grossan, an ENT-otolaryngologist in Los Angeles points to the science of psychoneuroimmunology (the study of how the brain is connected to the immune system), asserting that it has been shown 'over and over again' that depression weakens your immune system, while happiness on the other hand has been shown to boost our body's resistance.

"'What's crazy is that just the physical act of smiling can make a difference in building your immunity,' says Dr. Grossan. 'When you smile, the brain sees the muscle [activity] and assumes that humor is happening.'

"In a sense, the brain is a sucker for a grin. It doesn't bother to sort out whether you're smiling because you're genuinely joyous, or because you're just pretending."

Fascinating, isn't it? You can easily trick your brain into thinking that you are happy just by smiling, and your mood and body are rewarded in the process.

But you can do something that is even better than tricking your brain into thinking that you are happy. You can, instead, make a conscious decision to be happier. How do you do this? By focusing more on reasons you have to be happy, and then that smile will come naturally and will be a permanent part of your mug. (Why do I, at times, throw in an unexpected and somewhat silly word like "mug"? It makes me smile, and in the process, I'm trying to give you something to smile about too. Unexpected words can be very funny and they can generate both laughter and similes. And a good laugh, and a good smile, are like gold to our bodies and minds!)

This process starts with being more appreciative for what you have. It's almost like deciding that what you have is more valuable than what you had previously given it credit for. Doing that makes you rich. The value of everything you own, including your relationships with others, increases just because of that decision in your mind. You dig a little deeper to find more value in those things.

That's not an encouragement to lie to yourself with empty pep talks. But really take a look at some of the things you have. Do you live in a pretty area? Be thankful for that; appreciate it. Do you have one or more very good and trusted friends? Be appreciative for them, and let them know how you feel. Do you have access to good food? That's definitely something to be thankful for. Do you own a vehicle? If so, do you remember what it was like to get around when you were young and didn't have a vehicle? That's something to be thankful for too, and a reason to smile.

An appreciative attitude works wonders in a marriage. If you begin to focus more on the good qualities of your mate, you will have upgraded the status of your mate, and your marriage, in your conscious mind. Nothing has changed, but to you it is a reality. And such thinking will only, indeed, make your marriage even better.

One of the most beautiful things about smiles is that they come right back to you. Chances are good that when you smile at people, they will respond with their own pearly gift. And the beauty of this is that it doesn't even cost you a cent.

To close this chapter, let's revisit that wonderful article mentioned earlier with one more quote from Nicole Spector. She wrote: "Science has shown that the mere act of smiling can lift your mood, lower stress, boost your immune system and possibly even prolong your life." I'd call that a whole lot of benefit for zero cost and minimal effort. (If a pill could produce those effects, people would pay beaucoup bucks for it.)

And finally, I love the sentiment about the power of a smile from none other than the Uptown Girl herself, Christie Brinkley. She wrote: "A smile is an instant face lift and an instant mood lift." That thought, straight and simple, is so encouraging and meaningful, I'll allow it to conclude this book.

The very best of health, happiness, and well-being to you!

Index

adrenal hits, 24, 25
adrenaline, 24
aged cheese, 24
Aitken, Geoff, 101
almond milk, 44
Alyssa's Healthy Oatmeal Bites, 115
anthocyanins, 4
antibiotics, 13, 20
apples, 6
aquafaba, 28
Armstrong, Louis, 128
aspartame, 21
Atkins Diet, 42
author, not very bright, 101
avocado oil, 18
Ayers, Leonard, 62

back problems, 34
bacon, 16
Bacon, Sir Francis, 127
bacteria in mouth, 95
bacteria, healthy, 11
balanced meals, 9, 27, 37
banana test, 13
bank account, 127
Basketball Hall of Fame, 91, 92
bathroom scale, 35
beans, 17, 50
beans, white, 28

beat yourself up, don't, 122
Beattie, Melody, 119
beauty sleep, 81
beavers' anal glands (grossness alert), 20
Beckala, 98
beef, 54, 55
beef, grass-fed, 55
beef, grass-finished, 55
Berlin, Irving, 78
berries, 28
beta carotene, 4
BHA, 20
BHT, 20, 21
big business, 20
Big Dipper, 70
blender, 44
blender, high-speed, 44, 45
Blendtec, 44
blood pressure, 15, 88, 118
blood pressure, high, 34
blood sugar, 9, 27, 31, 77
blowing off steam, 116
blue light, 86
body temperature, 88
body weight, 77
body weight, use tape measure, 74
Bonahoom, Dr. Ronald, 100
Bradley, Bill, 91
brain, 15, 29, 31, 67

brain (a sucker for a grin), 129
brain exercise for senior citizens, 72
brain fog, 24
brain-teasing questions, 70
breakfast, 27
breakfast, when to eat, 28
Breatherian movement, 126
Brinkley, Christie, 130
Broken Heart: The Medical Consequences of Loneliness, The, 108
Brooks, Wiley, 126
Brown, Brené, 110
brushing teeth, rinsing well, 96
Bubbie's brand, 12
Bunker, Archie, 88
buttermilk, 12

cancer, 20, 34
carbohydrate cycling, 30
carbohydrates, natural, 17
carbohydrates, refined, 16
carbohydrates, slowed absorption of, 8
carob powder, 28
carrots, 16
Carter, Jimmy, 102
Carter, Rosalynn, 102
cartoons, 67
cartoons, written while asleep, 87

cashew milk, 44
cashews, 32
Centers for Disease Control and Prevention, 73
cesspools, and flossing, 96
cheating on diet, 38
checkers, 67
chemicals in food, 19, 35, 93
chess, 67
chewing food, 31, 33, 34, 40, 46, 97
chia seeds, 45
chicken, free-range, 53
chicken, organic, 53
chlorine, 11
chlorophyll, 4
chocolate, 25
cholesterol, high, 34
Chopin, Frédéric, 110
Christianson, Dr. Alan, 28, 40, 42
circadian rhythms, 78, 80, 85, 88, 89
clean your plate, 33
coconut milk, 12
constipation, 11
cortisol, 24, 30, 88, 125
cultured foods, 9

dairy, 12, 23
dairy products, 54
Darryl Stewart Wellness, 109
Day, Doris, 78
DeCelles, Emilee, 66

decision fatigue, 90
deep fried foods, 18, 22, 113
depression, 15, 79
diabetes, 15, 34, 114
diarrhea, 11
dietary blowouts, 38
dietary fat, 43
digestion, 11, 29, 31, 32, 40
digestive disorders, 34
digestive system, 11, 31, 33, 95
Donvito, Tina, 15, 16
dreams, 29
drink solids, chew liquids, 33

early death, 34
Earth, 6, 88, 125
Earth, a perfect match, 43
eating away from home, 38
eating slowly, 37
Edison, Thomas, 81
eggs, 23, 53
eggs, brown versus white, 54
eggs, Eggland's Best, 53
electric blanket, 111, 112
electric fields, 112
endorphins, 101, 128
enzymes, 9
Eschbacher, Roger, 102
EVOO, 7, 18, 50
exercise, 59
exercise, cardio, 59, 60
exercise, lifting for senior citizens, 65

exercise, lifting on consecutive days, 64
exercise, play, 66
exercise, resistance, 59
exercise, stretching, 59
exercise, weight repetitions, 63, 65
exercise, weight sets, 63
exercise, while listening to music, 61
exhaustion, 34

fad diets, 42
farming methods, 20
fast food restaurants, 113
fasting, 39
fasting, alternative, 40
fasting, burning muscle, 39
fasting, emergency mode, 39
fat loss (in specific areas?), 76
fats, 8, 18
fats, saturated, 19
fats, trans, 19
fatty liver, 41
fatty liver disease, 15
fermented foods, 12
financial problems, 34
fish, 52
fish, canned, 52
fish, smelling before buying, 95
flax seeds, 45
fluoride, 11, 96
food allergies, 23, 35

Food Babe, 20, 21
Food Babe Way, The, 20
Food Hunger Chart, 36
food industry, 21
food sensitivities, 35
football, 66
forgiveness, 118
Franklin, Benjamin, 90, 106
French fries, 17, 20
friend, how to be one, 109
friends, 130
fruit, 17, 28, 49

Garland, Judy, 78
gauss meter, 112
generosity, 120
gift giving, 109
Gifts of Imperfection: Let Go of Who You Think You're Supposed to Be and Embrace Who You Are, The, 110
glucono delta-lactone, 19
glycemic free, 17
Golan, Dr. Ralph, 79
grains, 50
grammatical boo-boos, 111
green banana flour, 28
Grier, Rosie, 99
grocery store, 115
Grossan, Dr. Murray, 129
growing old is not for sissies (quote), 66
GTOs, non-edible, 22
guilt, 34

gut health, 11

hamburgers, 93
Hari, Vani, 20, 21
health food stores, 113
health rebel, 94
heart, 4, 60
heart attack, 16
heart disease, 19, 34, 108, 114
heartburn, 34
high jumping, 105
high-carbohydrate breakfast, 27
high-fructose corn syrup, 15, 21, 55
high-protein breakfast, 27
hobbies, 99
honey, 17, 28
hormones, 20
hot dogs, 93
humor, 100
hunger, 15
hunger stop signal, 31, 34, 36, 37
Hutton, Betty, 78
hydration, 10
Hyman, Dr. Mark, 20

I Can't Get No Satisfaction, 87
I Got the Sun in the Mornin', 78
ice cream, 126

immune function, 11
insulin, 6, 15, 16, 31
intestinal system, 12
isometrics, 62
isotonics, 62
It Happened on Fifth Avenue, 107

Jabr, Ferris, 62
jet lag, 89
jogging, 61
Johnson, Rafer, 59
juice, 32
juice, raw, 9
juicer, 45
juicer, centrifugal, 45
juicer, masticating, 45
junk foods, 5, 21, 37

Karageorghis, Costas, 62
kefir, 12
keto diet, 8, 16, 42, 43
Keto Diet Damaged our Health: A Better Approach, The, 16, 42
kimchi, 12
Kindle books, 127
Klein, Rae, 101
Klein, Rebecca, 98
knee problems, 34
knowledge is power, 127
kombucha, 12
Krakovitz, Dr. Rob, 123

lard, 16
Lardie, Don, 110
laugh at yourself, 100
laughing, 100
Lectrofan, 86
legumes, 51, 52
Lennon, John, 87
lifespan, 15
light box, 79, 86
liver, 41
living foods, 9
love, 122
low-carb diet, 78
low-fat hysteria, 114
lungs, 60
lycopene, 4
Lynch, Dr. James J., 108

Macbeth, 81
macronutrients, 8, 9, 43
maple syrup, 17
marriage, and forgiveness, 118
Martin, Dean, 78
McCartney, Paul, 87
McKeever, Aloysius T., 107
McRaney, David, 117
meats, temperature cooking, 56
Mediterranean diet, 43, 47, 49
Mediterranean diet pyramid, 49
Mediterranean Diet pyramid, 48

Mediterranean region, 47
melatonin, 86, 88
Merman, Ethel, 78
Metabolism Reset Diet, 40
Metabolism Reset Diet, The, 41
metabolism, strong, 41
metabolism, weak, 41
Mexican fast food, 22
micronutrients, 43
microorganisms, 11
Microsoft Word, 90
milk, grass-fed, 54
mobility, loss of, 34
moderate food intake, 35
monk fruit (lo han), 17, 28
mood ring, 102
mood swings, 34
moon, 70, 88
mouth, 31
MSG, 21
music's effect on exercise, 62

natural foods, 42
natural foods, enjoying, 5
negative thinking, 105
night workers, 89
Ninja, 44
North Star, 70
Nutribullet, 44
nutrient absorption, 11
nuts, 9, 51
nuts and seeds, rancid, 51

obesity, 33, 34, 114

oils, hydrogenation, 7
Oldways, 48
olive oil, 9, 50
olive oil, extra virgin, 7, 18, 50
Omega juicer, 45
Opie (the neighbor's cat), 124
optical illusions, 71
oral health, 95
organic foods, 13, 35
overeating, 29, 31, 33, 35
overweight, 73

passive entertainment, 99
pathogens, 11
patience, 122
Payne, Grant, 113
peace, 116
peacemaker, 116
Peale, Norman Vincent, 106
peanuts, 23, 51
Pensacola, Florida, 71
perfectionism, 109, 110
Pet Rocks, 93
Phillips, Betty, 128
pickled vegetables, 12
plastics, 20
polar bears, 70
pork, 55
positive thinking, 105
poultry, 52
Power of Positive Thinking, The, 106
pre-sleep routine, 85

Pritikin Diet, 19, 42
probiotic count, 12
probiotic supplements, 12
probiotics, 11, 12
protein bars, 114, 115
protein powder, 45
protein shake, 28
pulp, 32, 45
pulse, 88
puzzles, 99

quinoa, 51

Rae Rae, 101
rain guards, 100
rainbow, 3
rainbow's colors of foods, 3
rat race, 124
raw foods, 9
Raw Foods Only Diet, 42
raw vegetables, 45
Reader's Digest, 15, 96
reading, 67
reading health books, 126
reality, 91
reddit, 73
refined carbohydrates, 15, 16
regular schedule (keeping), 87
relaxing, 47
resistant starch, 28, 45
Richards, Keith, 87
Rolling Stones, 87
Roseto, Pennsylvania, 107

Rosie Greer's Needlepoint for Men, 99
rowing, 61
running, 61

SAD (seasonal affective disorder), 79
saliva, 32
satiation signal, 31
sauerkraut, 12
Schaef, Anne Wilson, 109
Scientific American, 62
seafood, 52
seeds, 9, 51
self-esteem, low, 34
serotonin, 128
Shakespeare, William, 81
Shaw, Jeff, 102
shellfish, 23
Silly Putty (in food), 20
skin disorders, 12
sleep, 29
sleep apnea, 34
sleep compared to food, 84
sleep cycles, 10, 81
sleep debt, 81
sleep spindles, 83
sleep, bedroom cool, 86
sleep, bedroom dark, 86
sleep, non-REM, 82
sleep, poor quality, 85
sleep, REM, 82, 83, 84
sleep, stage one, 82
sleep, stage three, 83

sleep, stage two, 83
smiling, 120, 128, 129
smoothies, 44
snacking, 29
social issues, 34
soda, 20
sodium carboxymethyl cellulose, 19
solar eclipse, 71
soup, 9, 44
sourdough bread, 12
South Beach Diet, 42
soy milk, 12
Spector, Nicole, 129, 130
spirulina, 45
sprouted foods, 9
stair climbing, 61
stevia, 17, 28
Stivic, Mike "Meathead", 88
stomach, 31
stretching, 60
stretching, don't bounce, 59
stroke, 16, 34
sucralose, 21
Sudoku, 67, 101
Sudoku, cheap plug for my book, 72
Sudoku: Its Power Unleashed, 72
sugar, 15, 16, 55, 97, 114
sun, 88
sun, morning, 78
sun/moon comparison, 70
sweets, 55

swimming, 61

talk test, 61
tap water, 10
teeth, 15, 31
tennis, 72
thankfulness, 118
thirst (obey it), 11
Thompson, Ellen, 121
Thompson, Robert, 120
toxins, 20
trans fat, 22
treadmill walking, 61
triglycerides, 16
typos, 111

U.S. News and World Report, 47
University of Oklahoma, 108
urinary tract infections (UTIs), 12

Vale, Oregon, 71
vegan diet, 55
vegetables, 16, 50, 56
vegetables, non-starchy, 8
vegetarian diet, 55
venting anger, 116, 117
vitamin D, 79, 80
vitamin D, skin absorbtion, 80
Vitamix, 44

waist-height chart, 75

walking, 61
Washington Post, 73, 76
water, 10, 56
water bottle, 10
water, density while freezing, 70
water, how much to drink, 10
water, reverse osmosis filtering system, 11
we are what we eat (saying), 21
weight loss, 40
Wentz, Izabella, 94
wheat, 23
wheat grass, 45
Wheaties, 126
whispers (minor health issues), 123
white flour, 15, 113
white noise machine, 86
white sugar, 15, 113
Whole Foods, 44
Wilkinson, Bud, 66
window flaps, 100
Wolf, Dr. Stewart, 107

Xylitol, 17, 28

yoga mat softeners (in food), 20
yogurt, 12
You Are Not So Smart, 117

Other Books by David Klein

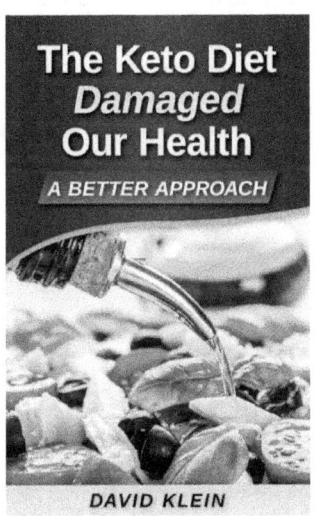

The Keto Diet Damaged Our Health: A Better Approach, is a thorough analysis of the ketogenic diet, which is now hugely popular. Many have lost weight by means of the keto. Does this mean that the keto diet is a healthy, nutritionally and medically sound diet, and that by going keto you'll be improving your health?

No. In fact, quite the opposite is true. The keto diet violates many time-tested and well-established rules and principles of nutrition and sound health. People who advocate the keto diet seem to think that no one ever lost a pound, let alone thirty or more, with any other method than keto. That's simply not true.

The U.S. News and World Report assembles a team of nutritional and medical experts each year, and then releases an evaluation of dozens of the world's most popular diets, and it ranks them by effectiveness according to several sub-categories. In 2017, the keto diet didn't even crack the top 10 diets for weight loss, and it came in dead last in overall diet for good health. Not exactly a stunning recommendation.

The keto diet is a medical trick on the body. And like the rest of us, the body does not like to be tricked, and it will rebel, making the keto dieter at risk of many serious medical problems.

Any diet that allows unlimited fat, including saturated fat, as well as chemicals in food and forbids or severely restricts healthful, power-packed nutritional foods like carrots is unsound. I offer a much better way to lose weight and get healthy. And not coincidentally, it's by following the same principles of nutrition in the book you are reading now.

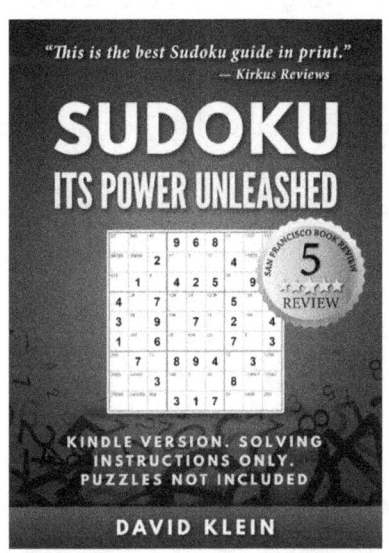

Sudoku: It's Power Unleashed, is the first of what I hope to be many Sudoku books. *Named "the best Sudoku guide in print" by Kirkus Reviews in January 2017*, the strength of this book is indeed the instruction. Learn to use many Sudoku solving methods, from the simple Only Candidate and Naked Twins, to the complex X-Wings, Y-Wings, Swordfish, and Unique Rectangles.

Five levels of puzzles are included, and candidates are provided with the puzzles, so that you can play using the most advanced methods and get to the fun and challenge of Sudoku right away.

Alphabet and Alphabet Hybrid puzzles are also a prominent feature of the book. Alphabet puzzles use letters instead of numbers, and several cells are shaded gray. When the puzzle is completed, the gray cells will spell something familiar, such as a location, book title, movie, person, food, and so on.

Alphabet Hybrid puzzles are played with numbers just like regular Sudoku puzzles, but a small conversion chart is provided where the numbers convert to letters. With a simple conversion of the shaded cells, the letters spell a location, book title, movie, person, food, and so on.

Additional hybrid puzzles include word guess, word scramble, brain playground, and math. For math puzzles, a mathematical equation is provided, with spaces for the numbers. Transfer the numbers from the shaded cells to the blanks and then complete the mathematical equation.

Note that the Kindle version of *Sudoku: Its Power Unleashed*, includes instruction only and does not include puzzles. It's not possible to play puzzles on a Kindle, which is strictly an electronic reader.

You can read the full review of *Sudoku: It's Power Unleashed*, by Kirkus Reviews. (They loved the book, awarding it a rare Kirkus star.) www.kirkusreviews.com/book-reviews/david-klein2/sudoku/

Furthermore, San Francisco Book Review awarded *Sudoku: It's Power Unleashed*, their highest rating of 5 stars.

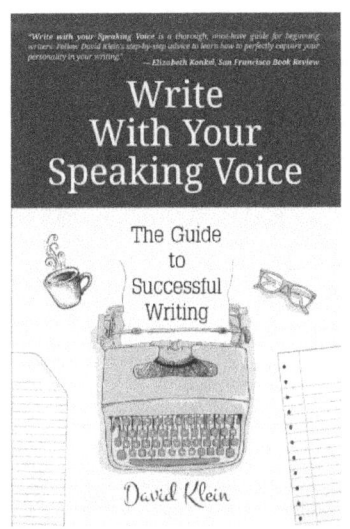

Write With Your Speaking Voice, is a writing guide for all who want to learn to write in a natural manner that matches their speaking voice. Flow-writing is explained, which allows the pattern of natural speech that flows from a speaker's mouth to instead flow to the keyboard or pen. Same speaker's patterns; same speaker's rhythms. Using your natural voice makes your writing effective; it will sound like your unique voice; it will sound like you.

Chapter titles include: Becoming a Skilled Writer, Capture Your Style of Speech, Flow-writing, Music—The Rhythm of Your Writing, Your Writing Voice, What to Write, When to Write, Writer's Block—Or Not Writer's Block, Humor, Personality, "Rules" to Put to Rest, Read Your Work Aloud, Tricky Word Choices, Self-Publishing, The Quote Collection, and many others.

Elizabeth Konkel, of the San Francisco Book Review, wrote: "*Write with your Speaking Voice* is a thorough, must-have guide for beginning writers. Follow David Klein's step-by-step advice to learn how to perfectly capture your personality in your writing."

San Francisco Book Review awarded *Write With Your Speaking Voice* their highest rating of 5 stars.

Write With Your Speaking Voice is available in Kindle and print editions.

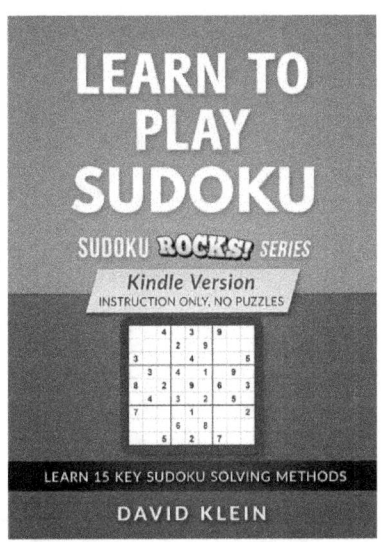

Learn to Play Sudoku rocks. It's loaded with puzzles, more than 500 of them, and they are rated at eight different levels of difficulty, including ridiculously easy to mind-boggling difficult—which are among the hardest puzzles in the world. With more than 40 pages of instruction, you'll learn to solve Sudoku puzzles more efficiently, and thus you'll enjoy playing Sudoku more and will be able to solve higher-level puzzles. (Puzzles are included in the print version only. Kindle books do not have puzzles because you can't play Sudoku on a Kindle, which is merely an electronic reader.)

Final Thoughts

I hope you have enjoyed reading this book and have learned valuable information that can help you live a healthier life.

If you like this book, please refer to chapter 47 and consider writing a review on Amazon. If you don't like this book, please refer to chapter 45.

David

www.ingramcontent.com/pod-product-compliance
Lightning Source LLC
Chambersburg PA
CBHW070231180526
45158CB00001BA/337